# The Hospital Admitting Department

American Hospital Association
840 North Lake Shore Drive
Chicago, Illinois 60611

Library of Congress Cataloging in Publication Data

American Hospital Association.
    The hospital admitting department.

    Bibliography: p.
    Includes index.
    1. Hospitals—Admission and discharge.  I.  Title.
RA971.8.A5   1976              658.7'28              76-54284
ISBN   0-87258-200-0

AHA catalog no. 004155

Printed in the U.S.A.
11M-1/77-5380
1M-11/81-7877
700-9/83-30861

# Contents

# List of Figures

# Preface

In 1952, the American Hospital Association first published *Manual of Admitting Practices and Procedures*, a comprehensive publication for hospital administrators and admitting department heads. The AHA Committee To Develop a Manual of Admitting Practices and Procedures had worked for several years to publish this long-needed, objective review of admitting policies and physical arrangements of hospital admitting offices, which vary considerably among institutions.

*The Hospital Admitting Department* is an extensive revision of that 1952 manual. The guidelines and considerations presented herein accept the challenging responsibility of the admitting department to create a satisfactory patient-hospital relationship during the admitting procedure. It includes 13 examples of forms and layouts and five appendixes. For those who are interested in further reading, there are lists of references.

Many persons have made this book possible. At the instigation of the AHA, a committee composed of AHA staff, admitting managers from several hospitals, and representatives of the National Association of Hospital Admitting Managers generated ideas on content and gave depth and direction to the project. Michael Kanter,* management consultant, Chicago Hospital Council, pulled the ideas together, explored their many dimensions, and wrote the manuscript, working in conjunction with J. Robert Pellar, director, and William A. MacFarlane, manager, respectively, of the council's Reimbursement Services division. Dorothy Saxner, Janet Plant, and Carole Bolster, of the AHA Books and Newsletters Department, coordinated the project, edited the manuscript, and guided it through the book production stages.

In addition, grateful acknowledgment is made to the following persons for their contributions: Marian Blankenship, director of medical record

---

*Mr. Kanter has since become a consultant with A. T. Kearney, Chicago.

and admitting services, Misericordia Hospital
Medical Center, Bronx, NY; John Collins, clinic
services coordinator, ambulatory care, Foster G.
McGaw Hospital, Loyola University, Maywood, IL;
John Coltella, admitting manager, Albert Merritt
Billings Hospital, Chicago; Ruth M. Grotzke, di-
rector of admissions and communications, St.
Francis Hospital, Blue Island, IL; Bernard Hiles,
director of admissions, Memorial Hospital of Du-
Page County, Elmhurst, IL; Arthur Isack, director
of ambulatory patient services, Foster G. McGaw
Hospital, Loyola University, Maywood, IL; Donald
M. Michels, assistant vice-president, Northwestern
Memorial Hospital, Chicago; and Phillip Moore,
director of ambulatory care, MacNeal Memorial
Hospital, Berwyn, IL.

# Introduction

The present-day admitting department reflects the changes of evolution. The marble counter that was common at the turn of the 20th century and later gave way to the small, austere admitting office has, in turn, been superseded by the friendly, pleasantly furnished department of today.

Accompanying these changes in the physical setting has been an increase in the responsibilities of the admitting staff. Basically, the department still governs the flow of patients and serves as a processing point through which all patients must pass. But its activities are being influenced increasingly by a number of external factors, such as professional liability, utilization review, and government-funded and other third-party reimbursement.

Today, admitting patients is only one of a number of functions performed. Admitting personnel are not merely clerks who register patients and assign them a room; they are persons vital to the successful operation of the hospital and must understand the relationships of their department to all other departments. In their position they can help the hospital to carry out a sound public relations program in the community, inasmuch as patients, relatives, visitors, physicians, and other hospital personnel all have contact with them. They also play an important role in maintaining good relations between the medical staff and other hospital personnel. Thus, everyone's reaction to the hospital is affected by the manner in which he is treated by the admitting staff.

To be successful, admitting staff must be able to appraise and be sympathetic to the specific fears of patients within the short time allotted for the admitting interview. An alert admitting staff is skillful in recognizing the various concerns that plague incoming patients. For example, to help families overcome their apprehension about the cost of hospitalization, the staff must patiently and tactfully explain the procedure for handling hospital bills. The staff must be aware that children may have fears arising from their pending separation from home, toys, and familiar surroundings. The staff must realize that some patients who enter the hospital are embarrassed about the treatment their illness requires, that some resent the misfortune of hospitalization, that some have anxiety arising from fear that the physician will discover an incurable disease, and that some are horrified at the prospect of an operation. Occasionally, the admitting staff encounters persons who are convinced that the hospital "experiments" on patients and who are therefore reluctant to place themselves in its care.

Patients' various fears and anxieties make it necessary for the admitting staff to be sympathetic to their feelings, yet at the same time the staff must perform its work efficiently. This task has become increasingly difficult with the complexity of patient information requirements; financial, demographic, and medical information is required to adequately fulfill hospitals' needs.

In order to carry out the department's functions properly, admitting personnel must:

• Determine the eligibility, number, and types of patients to be admitted to the hospital, in accordance with the policies and regulations established by the governing board, administration, and outside agencies

• Admit patients promptly and in an orderly manner to the various services of the hospital

• Maintain accurate records of patients awaiting admission and those already in the hospital

• Inspire in patients a feeling of trust and friendship by admitting them efficiently and graciously

The key to the success of the admitting department is its manager. In addition to possessing general managerial skills, this person must understand the importance of the department to the patient's overall well-being. The admitting manager must be able to combine sound administrative and operational skills with a sympathetic and compassionate concern for the patient, as well as possess a sensitivity to the vital role the hospital plays in meeting the health care needs of the community.

As a result of its increasing scope and complexity, the admitting department has become a crucial element in the hospital, and its operation is too complex to be simply dismissed as "another administrative detail." Admitting is, indeed, a major function in any hospital, and it warrants the attention of all those charged with administration and management of the institution. This book's intended audience, therefore, is the hospital administrator and assistant administrator, as well as the admitting manager and others responsible for management of the admitting function.

This book has been written as a guide. It is a general discussion of overall admitting considerations, rather than a detailed procedure manual. It should prove valuable as a means of reviewing responsibilities, functions, and procedures.

Not all of the activities outlined in the book are carried out in all admitting departments. Therefore, the portions that apply should be used as a means of assessment and evaluation for the individual hospital. Depending on the size and organization of the hospital, some of the admitting activities discussed may be handled by individuals who have other assignments. However, it is necessary that these activities be performed, even in hospitals not large enough to have a separate admitting department. Persons delegated the admitting responsibilities must be aware of all operational considerations, even though they devote only part of their time to this function.

With the increasing emphasis on ambulatory care, many hospitals have incorporated the ambulatory care registration function within the admitting department. This activity is playing an increasingly important role in the admitting manager's duties, and therefore it is addressed in this book. However, because of space limitations, a less detailed discussion of ambulatory care registration is presented than of inpatient admission. Primary aspects of inpatient admission are discussed in detail in chapters 1 through 6:

Chapter 1, Policies
Chapter 2, Organization and Personnel
Chapter 3, Functions and Procedures
Chapter 4, Legal Considerations
Chapter 5, Physical Characteristics
Chapter 6, Systems and Equipment

Chapter 7 is devoted to ambulatory care registration.

Patients' first impressions of hospitals remain with them and condition their feelings throughout their entire stay. It is therefore essential that satisfactory patient-hospital relationships be created during the admitting interview. This is the challenging responsibility of the admitting department. The main concern of the department is with incoming patients as human beings. All other considerations, though vital to hospital operations, are of secondary importance.

# chapter 1
# Policies

## POLICY FORMULATION

The admission of patients into a hospital occurs 24 hours a day, 365 days a year, in accordance with policies that reflect the governing board's philosophy of the role of the hospital as a community agency. The admitting staff works within the framework of these policies and the organizational pattern of the hospital. Properly developed policies ensure propriety and uniformity in the handling of patients and aid in the maintenance of good public relations.

### Existing Policies

The administrator must provide the admitting manager with the rules and regulations for implementing the policies of the governing board. Input for the formulation and establishment of admitting policies should be obtained from the medical staff, legal counsel, and other departments and parties as appropriate. All policies must be thoroughly reviewed on a regular basis to ensure compliance with all governmental and professional requirements, such as those of the Hill-Burton Act, Professional Standards Review Organizations, third-party payers, the Civil Rights Act, and the Joint Commission on Accreditation of Hospitals.

Policies should be in writing in order to ensure uniform application and consistent interpretation. Written policies are a guide in the performance of duties and facilitate the orientation and training of new employees. When policies are specifically spelled out in a written guide of rules and regulations, activities are expedited and the possibility of incorrect handling of patients through misunderstanding is greatly minimized. Written policies reduce error, and often spare the hospital embarrassment and the patient annoyance and even physical harm. Written rules also tend to eliminate tensions that might be detrimental to hospital-community relations, and they minimize the possibility of violation of governmental and professional requirements.

Failure to put all admitting policies in writing may result in:

- Inconsistent policies and resultant criticism of the hospital
- Personal interpretations of policies by admitting personnel
- Misunderstandings by the medical staff or hospital personnel about admitting policies
- Burdening administration with the necessity of making routine decisions
- Jeopardizing hospital accreditation or financial reimbursement
- Violations of legal requirements

### New Policies

New policies and revised policies should be established only after all of their probable effects have been explored. The administrator and the admitting manager should discuss proposed changes with the heads of other departments, because such changes may affect the routine of other departments.

After a new policy has been adopted or an existing one revised, the administrator, in consultation with the admitting manager, should establish a procedure to put it into effect. (Procedures are discussed in chapter 3.) A complete statement of the policy change should be distributed to hospital personnel and the medical staff. When necessary, other organizations should be notified; for example, if an admitting policy regarding the types of patients the hospital accepts is changed, the administrator should inform community agencies, so that they can cooperate.

## EXTERNAL FACTORS AFFECTING POLICIES

The number of external factors affecting hospital admitting policies has risen markedly in recent years. The health care field has seen a proliferation of legislation, professional standards, and third-party reimbursement regulations, all of which have to be considered in establishing admitting policies. A brief description of how some of these elements affect the admitting department follows.

### Hill-Burton Act

The Hill-Burton Act states that any hospital receiving funds appropriated under the act must provide a reasonable amount of services to persons unable to pay. Specific guidelines have been established to determine whether a hospital is meeting its obligations for provision of charitable care under the act.

One criterion for determining adherence is that the hospital certify that no person will be excluded from admission on the basis of inability to pay. If a hospital has received Hill-Burton funds, it is imperative that the admitting department know whether the hospital has elected this standard of compliance.

### Professional Standards Review Organizations

One of the provisions of Public Law 92-603 requires the establishment of Professional Standards Review Organizations to review the medical necessity for and the quality and level of institutional health care provided to beneficiaries under provisions of the Social Security Act. The common term for this process is utilization review.

A PSRO is a local organization of physicians responsible for the review of professional activities and the final pay/no pay decisions for patient care services delivered under federally funded health insurance programs in the PSRO's designated area. PSRO activities include concurrent review of admissions and continued patient stays; retrospective medical care evaluation studies; and analysis of provider (hospital), practitioner, and patient profiles. These activities can be carried out by the PSRO or can be delegated to hospitals.

PSRO activities have implications for admitting policies. Early initiation of discharge planning is essential in the concurrent review process in order to ensure that patients' health care needs continue to be met when the review process determines that an acute care bed is no longer medically necessary.

The admitting staff must be knowledgeable about the basic intent of the utilization review program in order that unnecessary admissions will be reduced and treatment of patients at an appropriate level will be ensured. The admitting staff must understand its role in ensuring compliance with the admitting criteria and standards established by the local PSRO. However, the admitting staff must also be aware that it has no authority or grounds for questioning or denying an admission authorized by a medical staff member in good standing.

The American Hospital Association's policy statement regarding utilization review and medical audit constitutes appendix A.

### Third-Party Reimbursement

In addition to the utilization review and PSRO requirements for third-party reimbursement, third-party payers require that they be notified of admissions, that benefits be verified, and that certain statistical and financial reports be made.

### Civil Rights Act

Discrimination and segregation on the basis of race, color, or national origin are prohibited by the Civil Rights Act of 1964, as amended. Race, color, or national origin cannot be used as a basis for denying admission or treatment of patients or for segregating them once they have been admitted. The Department of Health, Education, and Welfare has established guidelines prohibiting such discrimination and segregation by hospitals that receive funds under any programs supported by HEW.

### Joint Commission on Accreditation of Hospitals

The Joint Commission on Accreditation of Hospitals does not have a set of standards specifically for the admitting department, but certain of its standards have implications for admitting policies. The JCAH stipulates that inpatient medical records include a provisional diagnosis for each patient admitted. Therefore, it is useful for the admitting staff to understand the differences among the terms *diagnosis, symptom, diagnostic procedure,* and *surgical procedure.*

The JCAH also requires that "adequate appraisal, and advice or initial treatment, shall be rendered to any ill or injured person who presents himself at the hospital," even if the hospital refers all emergency patients to other institutions. (See Emergency Services, Standard I and its interpretation, *Accreditation Manual for Hospitals,* 1973.)

Hospitals are also required to have written plans for the "proper and timely care of casualties arising from both external and internal disasters, and shall periodically rehearse these plans." (See Environmental Services, Standard V, *Accreditation Manual for Hospitals,* 1973.) The hospital's disaster plan should take into consideration how inpatient admitting and discharge procedures should be modified during a disaster.

### Legal Considerations

Hospitals should review state and local laws and regulations to determine what elements, if any, might affect admitting policies. The policies and recommendations of medical and hospital associations and insurance commissions, as well as local licensing and antidiscrimination laws and regulations, might have an impact on the operation of the admitting department. (Chapter 4 discusses legal considerations.)

## SPECIFIC POLICIES

### Basic Types of Admissions

Because the demand for hospital beds frequently exceeds the supply, it has become common practice for admitting purposes to classify patients on the basis of medical need. Patients suffering from the severest illness or injury have the highest priority for admission and are admitted to the first available beds. The three most frequently used categories are emergency, urgent, and elective:

- *Emergency.* Immediate threat to the patient's life or well-being exists. This situation warrants the highest admitting priority. All reasonable measures are taken to ensure this patient's immediate admission, including the displacement or discharge of another less ill patient or temporary admission to the emergency department or patient unit corridor.

- *Urgent.* Undue or prolonged delay in admission might threaten the patient's life or well-being. The patient is promptly called when a bed becomes available. Normally, such patients should be admitted within 24 to 48 hours.

- *Elective.* The health of the patient is not endangered by delayed admission. Such patients are usually scheduled several days to several weeks in advance of admission. In consideration of the patient, the hospital should make every effort to accommodate this patient's desired date of admission. However, when circumstances dictate, this category of admission can be deferred. Often, these patients are processed through a preadmission program in advance of admission. (See chapter 3.)

The hospital's medical staff must develop criteria to define these three categories. Local factors such as patient population, services available, and the basic role of the hospital enter into the determination of the criteria.

Care must be taken to ensure proper application and nonabuse of the classification policy. A mechanism of medical review by staff physicians can reduce the possibility of patients being classified as emergencies when medical circumstances do not warrant immediate treatment. The admitting physician could be required to justify his decision through such a process as a deterrent to misuse of the classification system. The system should also not be used as a device for preferential treatment. Simply because a patient has been classified as an elective admission should not mean that he or she is given low priority on the reservation list in favor of someone with more adequate financial means or influence in the community.

## Criteria for Admission

Although the trend and ultimate aim of general hospitals is to admit all types of patients requiring medical treatment, many hospitals do, in fact, restrict the types of patients admitted. Current legal thought indicates that a person has no general legal right to admission except under certain emergency circumstances.

General hospitals frequently exclude alcoholic, drug-addicted, psychiatric, contagious disease, and terminal patients from admission for long-term care, inasmuch as adequate facilities and specially trained personnel may not be available to treat these types of patients and to protect the other patients. However, emergency circumstances may require that such patients be admitted on a short-term basis until other, more suitable, arrangements can be made.

Some private hospitals limit admission to patients from a specific geographic area. Other hospitals are restricted by law or other regulations to accept only certain types of patients. Many state, city, and county hospitals can accept only those who live within and are residents of a given geographic area; these hospitals may provide only emergency care to all others.

Age and sex are also factors that limit admissions. This restriction is usually based on the accommodations that are available, although there are hospitals that specialize in treating patients of a specific age range or sex.

Restrictions on admissions could occur as a result of peak occupancy. The hospital should determine the maximum number of patients it can serve and should have policies for referring patients to other hospitals or for otherwise assisting them during times of maximum occupancy.

Another limitation on admission is financial in nature. Some hospitals expect full payment for all services that they perform. Others offer free services to patients unable to pay. Still others—possibly the great majority—do both; that is, they expect full payment for the most part but do provide some charity care. If the hospital's cash revenues are modest, the governing board must carefully consider its charity policy on the basis of resources and availability of alternative community agencies and in light of any Hill-Burton obligations it may have.

For many patients, the financial responsibility is borne by a group outside the hospital. The advent of government-funded medical insurance has substantially increased the availability of health care to the public. The advent of national health insurance could be an additional consideration. Thorough knowledge and understanding of the various governmental and social agencies that finance health care for requisites for a well-informed admitting staff.

## Referral of Ineligible Patients

When ineligible patients present themselves for admission, they may be referred elsewhere if their condition permits. Whenever possible, a medical opinion should be obtained to confirm that the transfer will not be injurious to the patient.

Admitting personnel should have thorough knowledge of the resources of the community in order to be able to refer these patients to appropriate community agencies. If the hospital has a social service department, the admitting manager should refer ineligible patients to that department.

## Admission of Children

A decision must be made as to whether children are admitted to pediatrics or to a general unit. Age is perhaps the easiest and most reliable determining factor; the age limit used varies from hospital to hospital. The stage of physical development is also frequently used to determine where children should be assigned in the hospital.

## Admission of Newborn Infants

The administrator, in conjunction with the medical record administrator, the admitting manager, and the financial officer, should decide whether or not newborn infants should be assigned an admission number for the records of the hospital. If they are, the admitting staff is responsible for assigning the number. If a number is not assigned, the record of the newborn infant is simply made a part of the mother's medical record. If this is done, and the baby remains in the hospital after the mother goes home, the baby is usually admitted formally and assigned a number, and a separate medical record is prepared.

## Admission of VIPs and Public Figures

Many hospitals prefer to make special provisions for the admission of VIPs and public figures. Much discretion should be exercised in handling these situations; a delicate and sometimes precarious balance between special treatment for these patients and fairness to the other patients must be maintained. Although some individuals do warrant special treatment because of their public standing, the hospital and the admitting department must be careful to ensure against accusations of favoritism.

At the same time, the hospital must consider the rights of the persons involved. All patients, no matter how well known, should be accorded the right to privacy in their medical care. (However, reporting of vital statistics and of contagious diseases is mandatory.) The admitting department should take extra care in receiving and responding to any inquiries about well-known personalities. Inquiries should be referred to the public relations department or the administration. Some public figures may choose to use an assumed name while in the hospital or to pay cash for treatment rather than divulge their real identity. The admitting department, in conjunction with administration and other appropriate departments, must develop policies for handling such situations.

## Special Admission Situations

Policy provisions must be made for contingency and unusual situations that might confront the admitting department. Disaster and mass casualty policies and plans, for example, should be established in conjunction with local agencies in order to adequately meet community needs under such circumstances. Consideration must be given to how the admitting department can best receive and process a sizable number of casualties requiring admission at one time. Other contingency situations that require admitting policies are those involving police escorts, persons dead on arrival (DOAs), "bedside admissions," deaths in the admitting department, incomplete admissions because of insufficient information, cancelled admissions, and parents or relatives who wish to stay with the patient.

The policies developed by the admitting manager and the administrator for handling such situations must be consistent with the hospital's general policies. Although these situations do not occur frequently, the prudent administrator and manager will ensure that adequate policies and plans to handle them have been developed and disseminated and that admitting personnel are properly trained to implement the plans. These provisions could determine in large measure how successful the admitting program, and ultimately the hospital, is in meeting the health care needs of the community under unusual or adverse conditions.

The admitting department should have specific policies and plans to accommodate each foreseeable type of contingency. Checklists, exercises, and emergency procedure manuals should be developed as a means to properly train admitting staff in various disaster and unusual situations.

## Times for Admission and Discharge

The admitting department, in conjunction with administration, must establish times for routine admissions and discharges. Normally, it is desirable to encourage discharges during the morning and reserve the afternoon and early evening for admissions. This approach is especially applicable during high-occupancy periods, as it is essential for the admitting staff to know which beds have become available prior to assigning beds to incoming admissions.

Naturally, there are frequent exceptions to the normal admission and discharge hours. Emergency and urgent admissions occur at all times. Likewise, unusual circumstances necessitate discharge or interhospital transfer of patients at odd hours. Therefore, there must be policies for such exigencies.

Measures can be undertaken to encourage compliance with the desired admission and discharge hours. For example, nonemergency patients could be required to wait if they arrive at other than their assigned admission time, or an additional charge could be assessed to patients who leave the hospital after the stipulated discharge time. Such policies should be in accord with the general policies of the hospital.

## Admitting Privileges

The governing board has the ultimate authority and responsibility for granting admitting privileges to the medical staff. However, when considering an applicant, it can accept as its own the recommendations of the medical staff and the selection criteria established in the medical staff bylaws.

Likewise, the board must approve all suspensions, withdrawals, or limitations of privileges. Again, this can be done by adoption of medical staff recommendations and standards.

The admitting department must be aware of the privileges of each physician associated with the hospital in order to comply with the board's needs and desires. The maintenance of adequate patient care and of smooth administrative functioning requires that the admitting staff be informed about medical staff admitting privileges as a means of adherence to the governing board's determinations.

### Referral of Unassigned Patients

Occasionally, a patient seeks admission to the hospital on his own initiative. This person will not have been referred by a physician; he comes for care electively or as an emergency patient. To aid the admitting manager, the hospital should have policies for assigning such patients to medical staff members.

It is desirable to let the patient make his own choice from a list of staff physicians. The admitting department should therefore have a current list of staff physicians. If the patient is not interested in or capable of choosing his staff doctor, the decision should be made for him. How should this choice be made? If the hospital has a loosely organized medical staff, these patients usually are assigned by rotation of the entire staff. If there is rigid staff departmentalization, these patients might be assigned to physicians by rotation within the clinical department. Regardless of the method of assignment, the admitting staff must adhere strictly to the hospital's policies.

### Escort Service

The responsibility for escorting patients from the admitting department to their rooms may be assigned to the admitting staff, volunteers, nurses, or employees hired as escorts. Some hospitals provide escort service for patients being discharged. Hospitals may require that certain or all patients be transported in wheelchairs.

### Safeguarding of Patients' Valuables

Although patients should be encouraged not to bring large sums of money and other valuable items with them at the time of admission, suitable facilities should be provided for the safe storage of valuables. If possible, the person escorting the patient to the hospital should be requested to return the items to the patient's home.

If it does become necessary to store the patient's valuables, he should be informed that the hospital assumes no responsibility or liability for loss of or damage to items stored in or brought to patient care areas. All items should be stored in a suitable facility. Frequently, the cashier's area has a safe that can accommodate these items. The patient should be issued an itemized receipt for each valuable stored. At the time of discharge, each receipt should be signed by the patient and the person returning the items.

A release should be signed by the patient if he insists on storing valuables in his room.

### Patient Relations

The admitting department is a vital part of the hospital's overall public relations function. The hospital's preadmission and admission programs determine, to a large extent, patients' general impressions of and reactions to the hospital. Many seemingly minor features and aspects of the admitting process can become extremely important in forming favorable impressions.

It is recommended that the hospital develop a patient information brochure or booklet for distribution upon preadmission or admission. If it is not possible to distribute the brochure in the preadmission process, a letter explaining major hospital policies and assisting the patient with admission preparation could be mailed to him. Also, the brochure could be made available in clinics and doctors' offices. Any literature providing the patient with information about the hospital's operations, activities, policies, and procedures is helpful in alleviating anxiety and informing a patient of how he can best adhere to established hospital regulations. Such literature also serves to reduce the admitting department's task of verbal explanation.

Many hospitals have a patient representative program. Although the concept and the scope of these programs vary, the basic philosophy is to provide patients with one key person to handle all questions, problems, or complaints regarding their care and related administrative matters. The patient representative's functions may encompass some of the admitting staff's plus others normally handled in related departments or not otherwise provided. Depending on the particular program, the patient representative might help with preadmission, admission, financial arrangements, discharge planning, transfer to another facility, and other administrative matters necessary to ensure proper attention to patients' needs.

The American Hospital Association has developed *A Patient's Bill of Rights* with the "expectation that observance of these rights will contribute to more effective patient care and greater satisfaction for the patient, his physician, and the hospital organization." The complete bill of rights is given in appendix B. For those hospitals that have adopted the bill, the admitting department not only should be familiar with and observe these rights but also should inform patients of them when appropriate, in order to ensure their observance.

## Data Collection

The information that the admitting staff collects from patients is determined by state administrative rules and regulations governing licensure of hospitals, requirements of accrediting agencies and third-party payers, and the hospital's own operating needs.

## Financial Considerations

An adequate health care program cannot be maintained without satisfactory financing, and the admitting department is usually the primary area responsible for gathering financial information from patients. For indigent patients, this function may be accomplished in conjunction with the social service department. Complete and accurate information must be obtained.

If the hospital is not completely supported through government or philanthropic means, patients must provide payment through their own resources or through third-party reimbursement. Oftentimes, the admitting department is responsible for verifying insurance benefits with the providers and for notifying the various third-party payers of admissions.

The department should obtain a signature of payment guarantee from all patients, no matter what their financial status. The statement should indicate that no matter what insurance coverage the patient possesses, he is ultimately responsible for payment of his bill if other sources fail. Obtaining this signature from all patients will avoid any unintended impressions of discrimination. If the patient possesses insurance coverage, a signature for assignment of the benefits to the hospital should be obtained.

Frequently, if the patient is to pay for the services himself or if insufficient insurance coverage is available, an advance deposit is requested. The administration, in conjunction with the financial department, must establish a policy regarding deposits. In order for the admitting staff to properly adhere to policy, there must be clear definitions of which patients require a deposit and how much the deposit should be. A scale of the amount to be collected should be established. The factors to be considered are type of accommodation required, estimated cost of stay, and the patient's ability to pay.

Any questions or disputes that the admitting staff is unable to resolve regarding deposits should be referred to the collection manager. Usually, credit arrangements are also handled by the collection manager.

## Consents

The admitting department is usually responsible for obtaining general consents for treatment. The general consent form covers all procedures that do not require a special consent form. Blood transfusions and routine laboratory, diagnostic, and medical treatment are included. Hospital personnel, the attending physician, his assistants, and any other physician called upon by the attending physician, are thereby provided protection. Figures 1 and 2, pages 10 and 11, contain examples of a general consent form.

A hospital policy must be established as to who is responsible for obtaining special consents. Frequently, the specialty service department or physician obtains such consents. It is recommended that the physician be responsible for obtaining special consents at the time the procedure is explained to the patient. In any event, written documentation demonstrating that the patient or his legal representative knowingly and expressly authorized the treatment or procedure is advantageous in the event the treatment is challenged at a later date.

A special consent form should be obtained for the following procedures:

- Major or minor surgery
- Anesthesia
- Nonsurgical procedures that involve more than a slight risk of harm to the patient or that involve the risk of a change in the patient's body structure
- Cobalt or x-ray therapy
- Electroshock therapy or psychiatric treatment
- Experimental procedures

## CONSENT UPON ADMISSION TO HOSPITAL AND MEDICAL TREATMENT

PATIENT:_____

DATE:_____ TIME:_____ A.M.
                                                          P.M.

1.  I (or _____ for _____)
knowing that I (or _____) am (is) suffering
from a condition requiring hospital care, do hereby voluntarily consent to such hospital care encompassing routine diagnostic procedures and medical treatment by Dr. _____, his
assistants, or his designees as is necessary in his judgment.

2.  I am aware that the practice of medicine and surgery is not an
exact science, and I acknowledge that no guarantees have been
made to me as to the result of treatments or examination in the
hospital.

3.  Check one:
_____A. I hereby authorize the _____
Hospital to preserve for scientific or teaching purposes or for use
in grafts upon living persons or otherwise dispose of the dismem-
bered tissues, parts, or organs resulting from the procedure authorized above.

_____B. I will be fully responsible for making other dis-
position arrangements. Removal of that part from the hospital will
be accomplished within 5 days after discharge; failure to remove
before 5 days have passed will constitute approval of disposition by
_____Hospital under (A).

4.  This form has been fully explained to me, and I certify that I
understand its contents.

_____         _____
        Witness                     Signature of patient
(If patient is unable to consent or is a minor, complete the
following:)
Patient (is a minor_____years of age) is unable to consent
because_____
_____
_____.

_____         _____
        Witness                  Closest relative or legal guardian

Figure 1.  Example of General Consent Form
Reprinted, with permission, from the *Hospital Law Manual*, second edition, published
by Aspen Systems Corporation.

# MEDICOLEGAL CONSENT UPON ADMISSION TO HOSPITAL
# FOR DIAGNOSIS AND TREATMENT

A.M.

DATE:_____TIME:_____P.M.

I, _____, am entering _____ Hospital voluntarily
for the purpose of diagnosis and medical treatment and do hereby consent to such diagnostic procedures
and hospital care and to such medical, x-ray, nuclear, and electrical treatment, laboratory tests, and blood
transfusions as may be deemed necessary by Dr. _____,
his assistants, or designees. I have been advised, and I agree, that during my stay in_____
_____Hospital I may be attended by doctors, including Dr. _____
and one or more attending staff doctors, residents, interns, and medical students, any one or more of whom
may carry out a part, or all, of my treatment either alone or with the permission and guidance of Dr._____
_____.

I am aware that the practice of medicine is not an exact science, and I acknowledge that no guarantees
have been made to me as to the result of diagnosis, treatments, tests, or examination in_____
Hospital.

I hereby authorize _____ Hospital to complete any insurance forms submitted to them in
connection with my hospitalization.

I agree that _____ Hospital shall not be liable or responsible for the loss or damage to
any articles or personal property, including glasses and dentures, retained by me in my room and that items
having a monetary value, unless placed by me for safekeeping, at the time of admission, in facilities provided without charge by _____ Hospital, shall remain my obligation and responsibility.

This form has been fully explained to me, and I certify that I understand its contents.

_____          _____
Witness                                                        Signature of patient

(If patient is unable to consent or is a minor, complete the following:)

☐ Patient named above is a minor _____ years of age.
☐ Patient named above is unable to sign because:

_____.

For this reason, I am signing on behalf of the patient named.

_____          _____
Witness                                                        Signature of closest relative or legal guardian

                                                              _____
                                                              Relationship of signer to patient

Figure 2. Example of General Consent Form
Reprinted with the permission of Mercy Hospital and Medical Center, Chicago.

- All other procedures, as determined by the medical staff, that require a specific explanation to the patient. Any doubts as to the necessity of obtaining a special consent should be resolved in favor of obtaining it.

Figure 3, page 13, contains an example of a special consent form.

A patient has a right to refuse medical treatment to the extent permitted by law and to be informed of the medical consequences of his action. In the event that a patient does refuse treatment, the hospital should protect itself by obtaining a written waiver of liability that is consistent with applicable state law. The admitting department and administration should be familiar with the American Hospital Association's statement *The Right of the Patient To Refuse Treatment* (appendix C) and with state regulations regarding refusal of treatment.

### Confidentiality and Release of Information

At the time of admission, the patient should sign an authorization for the release of medical information for insurance, medical, and other legitimate purposes. The patient's signature on this document authorizes the hospital to conduct its legitimate affairs involving the patient's medical information without exposing the hospital to accusations of breach of confidence.

It is recommended that a release of information form be highly specific as to what information is to be released, why and how the requested information will be used, and how long the release is in effect. The form should also contain protection against the secondary release of information without the patient's consent.

Unofficial or questionable inquiries into patient medical information must be handled with utmost care and discretion. Admitting personnel should not discuss a patient's case with unauthorized persons, or even with the patient. Any inquiries regarding a patient by persons whom the admitting staff does not know to have specific authorization should be referred to administration, public relations, or other appropriate departments.

### Releases

If a patient wishes to leave the hospital against his physician's advice, the hospital cannot detain him. (Exceptions are psychiatric patients and patients with a contagious disease.) However, the hospital should obtain assurance that the patient has been informed of the inadvisability of leaving

and should ask him to sign a release form. In this way, the hospital may relieve itself from responsibility for the actions of the patient.

If a patient is physically helpless or mentally incompetent, the hospital should have the person who is legally responsible for him sign a special form before the patient is released. Under no circumstances should such a patient be allowed to leave the hospital unescorted.

If the patient is a minor, the signature of a parent should be obtained.

The nursing department is usually responsible for obtaining signatures on releases, but sometimes this function is shared with the admitting department. The admitting staff should therefore understand all local laws and regulations governing the release of hospital patients.

### Bed Assignments

The paramount concern in regard to bed assignments is fair and equitable distribution of beds in accordance with the medical needs of the patient population. These needs are determined by administration and the medical staff. Barring genuine medical emergency, such secondary factors as service required, sex, age, and ability to pay may enter into the assignment of beds. However, religion, race, and ethnic or national origins should never play a role in bed assignment.

When the hospital is experiencing a low occupancy rate, patients should generally be served on a first-come, first-served basis. In high-occupancy periods, beds should be assigned in accordance with the priority system previously described: emergency, urgent, and elective admissions.

It is desirable to maintain as even an occupancy rate as possible without jeopardizing the welfare of the patients. In other words, no patient should be denied or deferred admission against medical advice simply to smooth the occupancy rate. However, it may be advantageous to schedule some elective admissions for normally low-occupancy periods. Typically, the beginning and middle of each week are high-occupancy periods, whereas the latter part of the week and the weekend are low-occupancy periods. Consideration can therefore be given to formulating an admitting policy that encourages elective admissions at the end of the week and on weekends if other factors do not preclude this possibility. An adjustment in schedules for the operating room and laboratory facilities may have to be made in conjunction with this policy. Naturally, coordi-

# SPECIAL CONSENT TO OPERATION
## OR OTHER PROCEDURE

PATIENT:_____ DATE:_____

TIME:_____ A.M.
                   P.M.

1. I hereby authorize Dr. _____ and/or such assistants as may be selected by him to treat the condition or conditions which appear indicated by the diagnostic studies already performed.
(Explain the nature of the condition and the need to treat such condition.)

_____ .

2. The procedure(s) necessary to treat my condition (has, have) been explained to me by Dr. _____, and I understand the nature of the procedure to be: _____
(A description of the procedure(s) in the language of laymen)

_____ .

3. It has been explained to me that, during the course of the operation, unforeseen conditions may be revealed that necessitate an extension of the original procedure(s) or different procedure(s) than those set forth in Paragraph 2. I therefore authorize and request that the above named surgeon, his assistants, or his designees perform such surgical procedures as are necessary and desirable in the exercise of professional judgment. The authority granted under this Paragraph 3 shall extend to treating all conditions that require treatment and are not known to Dr._____at the time the operation is commenced.

4. I have been made aware of certain risk(s) and consequences that are associated with the procedure(s) described in Paragraph 2. These are:
(A description of the risks and consequences that are involved in this particular procedure)

_____ .

5. I have also been informed there are other risks such as severe loss of blood, infection, cardiac arrest, etc., that are attendant to the performance of any surgical procedure. I am aware that the practice of medicine and surgery is not an exact science, and I acknowledge that no guarantees have been made to me concerning the results of the operation or procedure.

6. I consent to the administration of anesthesia to be applied by or under the direction and supervision of Dr. _____.

_____     _____
      Witness                       Signature of patient

(If patient is unable to sign or is a minor, complete the following:)
Patient (is a minor_____years of age) and is unable to sign because

_____ .

_____     _____
      Witness                 Closest relative or legal guardian

Figure 3. Example of Special Consent Form
Reprinted, with permission, from the *Hospital Law Manual*, second edition, published by Aspen Systems Corporation.

nation and consultation with the medical staff are vital to successful implementation of such an adjusted admitting schedule.

### Transfers within the Hospital

If it becomes necessary to move a patient from one accommodation to another, the admitting department should be authorized to carry out such action within existing regulations. For example, if a patient in a ward or a semiprivate bed should be moved to a private accommodation because of his medical condition, the admitting manager should be authorized to effect the transfer. Patients who often require private rooms are those with a mental condition, with a contagious disease, or in the terminal stage of an illness. All patient transfers should be approved by the attending physician and should be coordinated with the nursing staff and units involved.

If the information pamphlet for patients states that the hospital retains the right to transfer patients at its discretion, misunderstandings will be minimized.

Efforts should be made to minimize transfers that are requested simply for the patient's convenience, inasmuch as each transfer disrupts hospital routine. The labor and the communications required for a patient transfer are considerable. The simple task of moving a bed marker from one position to another initiates a chain of events that can be a burden to the hospital.

### Discharges and Transfers to Other Facilities

The admitting department should be informed of all scheduled discharges immediately. A pending discharge (discharge forecasting) system provides a basis for scheduling upcoming admissions on the basis of projected bed availability. At the actual time of discharge, the admitting department must be notified, so that a specific bed assignment can be made.

The admitting department may be involved in the coordination of a patient transfer to another institution, such as a special or an extended care facility. However, the primary responsibility for this function usually rests with the social service or the nursing department.

### Patient Leaves of Absence

Occasionally a patient requests permission to leave the hospital for a short period. Because the hospital runs the risk of being criticized if anything untoward happens to the patient while he is away, some hospitals discourage leaves of absence. Some hospitals permit leaves of absence if patients do not remain away overnight; otherwise they are discharged.

When a patient is permitted to leave, he should sign a form releasing the hospital from any liability for his action. Leaves should be permitted only when approved by medical opinion documented in the patient's medical record.

Consideration should be given to how to count such patients for census purposes. A Medicare provision requires that the day a patient begins a leave of absence be treated as a day of discharge and not be counted as an inpatient day unless the patient returns by midnight of the same day. The day the patient returns is treated as a day of admission and is counted as an inpatient day if the patient returns by midnight.

### Utilization Review

The federally mandated utilization review program (PSRO) markedly affects management of bed resources, as one of the intents of this program is to ensure that all hospital admissions (use of beds) are necessary. The admitting physician will possibly be subject to justification of admissions, although current provisions require justification on an exception basis only. The admitting staff and all others connected with admissions should be familiar with the basic provisions of this law, as well as the American Hospital Association's statement *Utilization Review and Medical Audit in the Health Care Institution* (appendix A).

### Disasters and Labor Stoppages

In the event of internal or external disasters or of work stoppages, the admitting department must have policies for assigning beds according to the greatest medical need and current capabilities of the hospital. It may be necessary to deny admission to or discharge patients with limited medical needs. In some instances, contingency beds must be made available to accommodate the temporarily excessive demand for beds. Such emergencies may necessitate policies concerning communication between the admitting and the public relations departments.

### Opening and Closing Beds

As the census and staffing of the hospital fluctuate, it may become necessary to open or close various patient care units. The admitting department usually does not have unilateral authority to open or close a unit. This decision must be made by the administration or possibly the board of directors, in consultation with the medical director of the unit. However, the admitting department should provide input for the decision and should be informed of the ultimate decision in order to implement it.

**Notification of New Admissions**

The admitting department plays an instrumental role in informing various departments of new admissions, and, in some hospitals, of discharges and inhouse transfers. As the initial point of contact with the patient, admitting is the logical department to serve in this capacity. Generally, all departments that serve patients directly or indirectly must be aware of their arrival, location, and departure. (This notification process and the departments to be notified are described in chapter 3.)

**Communication with Administration and the Medical Staff**

It is imperative that the admitting department maintain good communication with administration and medical staff, informing them of unusual situations. The advice and counsel of administration and the medical staff should be solicited on questions regarding admission, discharge, or transfer of a patient; the appropriateness of releasing information on a patient; unusual financial arrangements; and consents for or refusals of treatment. Also, the medical staff should be kept informed of pertinent policies and procedures, current hospital rates, occupancy statistics, desired advance notification times and hours of admission for elective patients, and reservation and discharge procedures.

Good communication between admitting, administration, and the medical staff minimizes misunderstandings and confusion and facilitates overall admitting operations. The need for constant communication cannot be overemphasized.

**Reports of Patients' Conditions**

Whether or not the admitting department has the responsibility for providing information about patients to their families and the public depends on the physical layout of the hospital and upon available personnel. If the hospital does not operate an information desk, the admitting department may have to perform this function. Because the admitting department has daily contact with nursing stations, it logically may serve as the information desk. Before placing this responsibility with the admitting department, however, the administrator should make certain that it will not interfere with the primary work of the department.

# References

American Hospital Association. *Hospital Medical Records: Guidelines for Their Use and the Release of Medical Information.* Chicago: AHA, 1972, pp. 4-9, 14-20.

_____. *Principles of Disaster Preparedness for Hospitals.* Chicago: AHA, 1971.

American Medical Record Association. *Public Law 92-603, PSRO.* Chicago: AMRA, 1973.

Hayt, E. *Law of Hospital, Physician and Patient.* 3rd ed. Berwyn, IL: Physicians' Record Co., 1972, pp. 83-158, 419-512, 573-88, 1057-1150.

Hospital Research and Educational Trust. *Guide for the Utilization Review Coordinator in a Quality Assurance Program.* Chicago: HRET, 1974.

Joint Commission on Accreditation of Hospitals. *Accreditation Manual for Hospitals.* 1970 ed., updated 1973. Chicago: JCAH, 1973.

MacEachern, M. *Hospital Organization and Management.* 3rd ed. Berwyn, IL: Physicians' Record Co., 1957, pp. 125-56.

University of Pittsburgh, Health Law Center. *Hospital Law Manual.* 2nd ed. Administrators' vols. 1 and 1A. Germantown, MD: Aspen Systems Corp., 1974, Admitting and Discharge sections 1-4, Governing Board section 5, Financial Management sections 1 and 8-10, Medical Staff sections 1-3.

chapter 2
# Organization and Personnel

## ORGANIZATION

The policies of the hospital as defined by the governing board and the administrator are directly reflected in the organization and staffing of the admitting department. Because of wide differences in hospital organization, no two admitting departments are identical. Their specific functions vary, being influenced by types of treatment for patients, medical and financial policies, number of beds, and location.

The number of beds may determine the degree to which the admitting function is specialized. In hospitals that have a small number of annual admissions, the job of admitting manager may be combined with other jobs. Because admitting policies are closely related to financial matters, the admitting manager often shares or fully assumes the financial responsibilities. Other jobs sometimes combined with that of admitting manager are assistant administrator, nursing director, medical record administrator, and social service director.

Such job combinations are found primarily in small hospitals, where the volume of admissions makes it impractical to have a department or person devoted to the admitting function on a full-time basis. However, a part-time admitting manager is rapidly becoming the exception. Because of the increased complexity of the admitting function and the increased demand for health care, most hospitals have at least one person, if not a department, devoted entirely to the admission of patients.

### Factors Governing Establishment of a Separate Admitting Department

The number of patients admitted and the time required to interview them are the main factors determining whether or not a separate admitting department is established. Hospitals dependent mainly upon patient revenue for income usually find that a full-time admitting department is justifiable.

The types of patients accepted are also a factor in the establishment of a separate admitting department. Hospitals treating primarily short-term, acutely ill patients have many more admissions per bed than hospitals treating long-term patients, such as mental, terminal, drug-addicted, and alcohol-addicted patients. Thus, acute-care hospitals usually require a full-time admitting manager, whereas long-term care hospitals often can manage with a part-time employee in that position.

### Lines of Authority

In establishing reporting responsibility and lines of authority for the admitting department, administration must consider where the emphasis of the admitting functions is to be placed. Is the greatest need to gather complete and accurate financial and insurance information; to deal with the medical, sociological, and psychological needs of patients during the admitting process; or to gather complete data for medical record purposes? The answer to this question may help to determine where to place the admitting department within the overall hospital organizational structure. For example, if the greatest need is to gather medical record data, the admitting manager could report to the head of the medical record department. It may be most appropriate to place admitting under an assistant administrator who has organizational responsibility for several of the departments that have direct contact with admitting.

### Relations with Other Departments and Services

The admitting department must maintain close contact with the following departments and services:

- *Medical records.* Admitting must notify the medical record department of admissions, so that previous medical records can be retrieved. Admitting originates the face sheet of the medical record, may obtain the signatures on release and consent forms, which are part of the medical record, and provides input for various statistics on the medical record. If the hospital utilizes a unit numbering system, the medical record department usually assigns the numbers.
- *Nursing.* Admitting must notify nurses' stations of incoming admissions, and the nursing department, in turn, must notify admitting of all patient transfers and discharges. Admitting originates the medical record, as already men-

tioned, and also makes up the patient's identification and imprinting plates.
- *Ambulatory care.* Procedures must be established for the admission of patients from outpatient and emergency services. Admitting may be responsible for the control of patient numbers in the ambulatory care areas. (See chapter 7 for a discussion of ambulatory care registration.)
- *Data processing.* Admitting is responsible for the input of data used in the billing and accounting systems. Various medical and statistical data used in computerized systems may also be provided by the admitting department, in order to generate such reports as a computerized census.
- *Ancillary departments.* If the hospital has a pre-admission testing program, admitting must coordinate test arrangements and provision of test results with appropriate ancillary departments, usually the laboratory and radiology. Many hospitals require a battery of tests at the actual time of admission, which admitting must coordinate with the appropriate departments. Admitting may also be responsible for autopsy arrangements with the pathology laboratory.
- *Public relations.* The admitting department usually does not assume responsibility for releasing patient information to unauthorized parties. When such inquiries are made to admitting, they should normally be referred to the public relations office for handling.
- *Business office.* The admitting department plays a key role in the financial systems of the hospital, as it gathers the necessary information for the billing and collection processes.
- *Social service.* Admitting may work with social service staff in making financial arrangements for indigent patients. Admitting may also be involved in the coordination of discharge planning for some patients.
- *Volunteers.* Admitting may coordinate escort services provided by volunteers.

## PERSONNEL

In large part, the admitting staff represents the hospital to the community. During the activities of a single day, admitting personnel may be in contact with more persons than any other hospital employees. The admitting staff talks to incoming patients, their relatives and friends, doctors, other hospital employees, police officers, and undertakers. Because the manner in which the staff carries out its duties significantly influences the community's opinion of the hospital, admitting personnel must exercise considerable tact in their relationships with these diverse groups. Particularly, the staff must be acutely sensitive to patients and their problems.

## Qualifications

Admitting personnel should be emotionally stable and mature. They should be able to maintain poise even under pressure. For example, it is difficult for an admitting staff member to remain courteous and diplomatic when physicians attempt to secure admission for their patients at a time of full occupancy. Surmounting the emotional tensions that arise in such situations and in relationships with so many persons continually proves a challenge for admitting personnel.

Admitting personnel should have a talent for evaluating people quickly and accurately. Furthermore, they should have the intelligence to acquire a working knowledge of medical terminology within a relatively short time, in order to be able to write an admitting diagnosis correctly.

Personal traits are also important. Admitting personnel should be pleasant and cheerful, in order to obtain the highest degree of cooperation when dealing with people. They should also be well groomed.

Because of the clerical nature of many admitting activities, most hospitals regard clerical skills, in addition to communication and human relations skills, as primary vocational requirements. The abilities to type rapidly and accurately, gather complete and accurate information, file and organize documents in a logical manner, and operate various types of office equipment are prerequisites to satisfactory job performance.

Admitting personnel come from various occupational backgrounds. Some hospitals prefer to use persons with a financial orientation, such as individuals with credit and collection experience. Other hospitals prefer to use nurses or social service workers, in an attempt to emphasize the patient care aspects of admitting. However, if there is a shortage of nurses or social workers, it is extravagant to use them in the admitting department, where their skills cannot be fully utilized. Instead, when their input is required, it can be made available in an advisory capacity.

Essential to the admitting department is the admitting manager. He must be able to combine sound administrative and operational skills with a sympathetic and compassionate concern for patients.

## Duties

The basic tasks of the admitting staff are controlling and arranging reservations, preadmissions, admissions, bed assignments, transfers, and discharges. Additional duties may be assigned as individual hospital circumstances require. (The duties of the admitting staff were described in terms of policy in chapter 1 and are discussed in terms of procedure in chapter 3.)

The job descriptions developed by the Department of Labor for an admitting officer and for an admitting clerk present the duties, traits, and experience necessary to perform in these capacities. They are shown in appendix F along with an AHA careers pamphlet on becoming an admitting officer. They are general in nature and must be modified for each hospital's operating environment.

## Orientation and Training

A formal training program should be developed for all new admitting personnel. It should consist of two major elements: orientation to the overall hospital and orientation to the admitting department. The policies and procedures of both the hospital and the department should be presented. Therefore, it is vital that a comprehensive, clearly written policy and procedure manual be available. This document serves as a training tool during orientation and as a convenient reference thereafter. The use of additional training devices, such as films, brochures, and lectures, is also desirable. However, nothing can supplant the experience gained from a well-planned and supervised on-the-job training program.

## Staffing

The admitting department functions 24 hours a day, 7 days a week, as the admission of emergency patients cannot be controlled or scheduled. Although the majority of admissions and discharges occur daily from 9 a.m. to 7 p.m., someone must be available at all times to handle unexpected admissions and discharges.

In large hospitals, the admitting department is staffed around the clock. Some hospitals may even require several persons on the evening and night shifts in order to perform duties not suitable for the day shift, such as manual compilation of the census, gathering of preadmission information, and preparation of patient folders for admissions scheduled for the following day.

In small hospitals, it may be sufficient to assign admitting responsibilities to another department during the evening and night. The nursing supervisor, the night administrator, the cashier, or the switchboard operator may assume this duty. If this is the case, the admitting manager should maintain close liaison with the designated individual to ensure that admitting procedures are properly carried out and to be kept apprised of any unusual occurrences.

An example of the organizational structure within the admitting department is shown in figure 4, page 21.

# References

American Medical Record Association and Greater Portland Admitting Officers Association. *Management Guide for Admitting Personnel.* Chicago: AMRA, 1975, pp. 3-5.

U.S. Department of Labor, Manpower Administration. *Job Descriptions and Organizational Analysis for Hospitals and Related Health Services.* rev. ed. Washington, DC: Government Printing Office, 1970, pp. 102-04, 115-16.

## ORGANIZATIONAL CHART

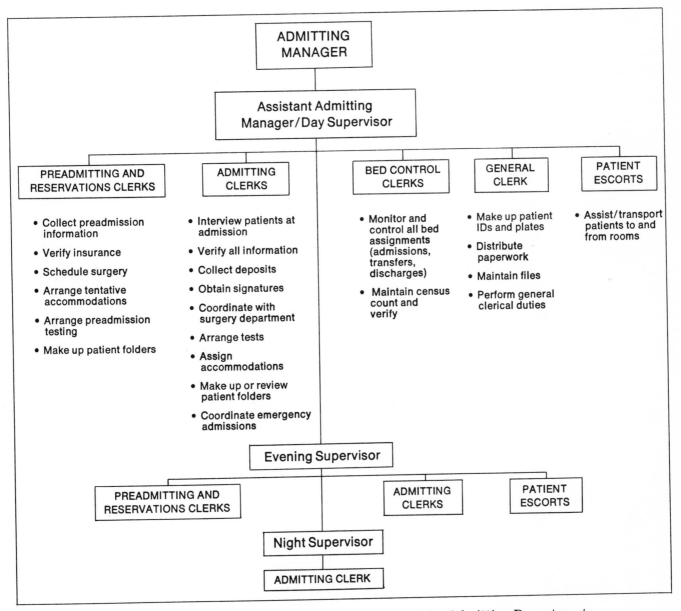

Figure 4.   Example of Organizational Structure of the Admitting Department

NOTE: This organization chart is not intended to depict the ideal admitting department; it merely illustrates the major functions and positions commonly found in the department. Many hospitals do not require this complex or large an organizational structure; small hospitals generally combine various admitting functions and positions.

# chapter 3

# *Functions and Procedures*

No department can function adequately without well-planned and well-designed procedures. This is as true for the admitting department as it is for the other departments in the hospital.

The systems and procedures used in the admitting department must support the objectives of placing each patient in the most suitable accommodation in accordance with his medical needs and collecting all patient data and information necessary for the provision and administration of health care.

An efficient admitting system has the following characteristics:

- It retains complete control over the initiation of all records relating to the admission of patients. This authority minimizes the number of copying errors.

- It notifies other departments of the hospital immediately upon the arrival of patients.

- It provides other departments with prompt notification of discharges and transfers.

- It maintains an accurate bed control system.

- It keeps complete and uniform records.

- It maintains specific procedures that govern the duties of all personnel who handle the admission, transfer, and discharge of patients.

- It provides patients and relatives of patients with an accurate and full explanation of pertinent hospital policies.

Admitting procedures, like policies, should be in writing to make sure operations run smoothly and to prevent misunderstandings. Before they are implemented, new procedures and changes in existing procedures should be discussed with the heads of other departments whose operations would be affected.

This chapter describes in general terms the basic functions of the admitting department and the procedures necessary to support them.

## PREADMISSION

An efficient preadmission system significantly facilitates and enhances the overall admitting program. A preadmission program applies primarily to elective admissions but also, at times, to urgent admissions.

Its advantages are numerous. It expedites the processing of admissions and thus reduces delays and the time required to place a patient in a bed. Hospital routines are less likely to be disrupted, because related departments are made aware of a patient's pending arrival sufficiently in advance so that necessary preparations can be made. The patient is more likely to be assigned to the most appropriate type of accommodation and clinical service, since requirements are known prior to arrival.

The basic elements of a preadmission system are as follows.

### Reservations

Several days to several weeks prior to actual admission, the attending physician notifies the admitting department that a patient will require admission. The admitting department should obtain as much relevant information as possible at that time. Generally, a reservation form can be used for this purpose.

The major information items to be collected are:

- Admitting physician's name.
- Patient's full name.
- Patient's full address and telephone number. If the patient does not have a telephone, a neighbor's or close relative's number should be obtained.
- Patient's age and sex.
- Physician's medical staff status: active, associate, or courtesy. (This information is available from the medical staff roster.) If a physician's admitting privileges have been suspended for any reason, admission is usually denied unless a genuine emergency exists.
- Room requirement and preference.
- Clinical service required.
- Patient financial information: Blue Cross/Blue Shield, Medicare, Medicaid, other government payments, commercial insurance, self-paying, Workmen's Compensation, charity, prepaid group program, or other.
- Specific surgical procedure, if required, and date.

- Admission classification: elective (usually), urgent (sometimes).
- Desired date of admission.
- Admitting diagnosis.

This information is stored in an appropriate filing system until the remaining preadmission information is gathered. A tickler file arranged by date of scheduled admission is a suitable means of storing this information. It enables access to the information when the admitting staff collects the remaining data.

### Additional Data Collection

The preadmission program allows for collection of most of the remaining information prior to the patient's arrival. In addition to the information obtained with the reservation, the admitting department must obtain more specific demographic, sociological, and insurance information.

The additional data can be collected by mail, telephone, or interview, depending on the lead time available and the type of patient population. If the lead time is several weeks and the people in the community generally respond adequately, mailing a preadmission form to the patient may suffice. However, if the lead time is only several days and adequate response cannot be expected, it may be necessary to conduct a preadmission interview via the telephone or when the patient comes to the hospital for his preadmission tests. An interview has the advantage of personalizing the process and allowing the patient to ask questions, but it is time-consuming for the staff.

Since the additional preadmission information is the same as that gathered during the normal admitting process, a standard admitting form (figure 7, page 32, discussed in more detail later in this chapter) can be used. It may be desirable to maintain patient folders containing all preadmission documents, including the patient treatment orders that many doctors write prior to admission. Such orders can be stored in the folders until the orders are forwarded to the patient unit. The folders can be filed according to scheduled admitting date. The same folder can thus be used to store all financial and related documents during the patient's stay and after.

### Insurance Verification

As part of the preadmission program, some admitting departments verify patients' commercial insurance and Workmen's Compensation benefits and prepare notices of admission for Blue Cross, Medicare, and Medicaid patients. If these procedures are accomplished prior to admission, confusion or embarrassment regarding a patient's financial coverage is minimized. Alternative financial arrangements can be made in advance of admission if the patient's coverage is not as comprehensive as originally anticipated.

In a program developed by the Chicago Hospital Council for standardizing and expediting the insurance verification and claims process, the participating hospitals use a standardized notification and claim form (figure 5, pages 26 and 27) for most of the major commercial insurers, who cooperate in honoring the form.

### Certification and Utilization Review

The preadmission program enables review and certification procedures to be conducted prior to the patient's admission. This is termed prospective review. The patient's admission and his projected medical treatment are certified as appropriate and necessary to ensure the best care for him and the best utilization of available health care resources on the basis of documentation supplied by the admitting physician. Prospective review can also aid the hospital in avoiding financial loss. Admitting provides the necessary input to the reviewing parties.

### Preadmission Testing

The reception and processing of patients are greatly facilitated if necessary diagnostic tests and procedures are conducted on an outpatient basis before admission. Preadmission testing eliminates delay at the time of admission and increases the probability of having test results available for the physician's review when the patient is admitted. The admitting department is usually involved in the scheduling and coordination of preadmission testing and receives completed test results for insertion in the patient's medical chart prior to his arrival in the patient unit.

### Surgery Scheduling

A preadmission program greatly improves coordination between admitting and the surgical suite. Necessary surgery facilities can be scheduled well in advance of the patient's anticipated admission date. This eases the burden on operating room facilities and allows for improved workload and staff scheduling. The admitting department must work closely with surgery personnel to properly coordinate this scheduling.

Some hospitals allow the admitting department to schedule surgery. The disadvantage of this approach, however, is that most admitting personnel are not sufficiently knowledgeable about the time required for various procedures and by various surgeons. It is generally more satisfactory to develop good rapport between admitting and surgery than to use this arrangement.

## ADMISSION

Admission of patients is the most vital part of the admitting department's operation. Whether or not there is a preadmission program, the admitting process must ensure that the patient is placed in a suitable bed and that all necessary information is obtained.

### Reception and Initial Contact

Chapter 1 described the basic policy considerations related to reception of and initial contact with patients. Essentially, the admitting staff is responsible for:

- Receiving the patient in a courteous and accommodating fashion.
- Determining his eligibility for admission in accordance with established hospital criteria.
- Ascertaining the patient's admitting classification: emergency, urgent, or elective.
- Ensuring that the patient has arrived on the correct date and at the correct time.
- Verifying that the physician's request for admission of the patient is in accord with his staff privileges.
- Ascertaining the clinical service required and the type of accommodation required or desired by the patient.
- Informing the patient of all pertinent hospital policies and of his rights. Distribute the hospital's patient information brochure.
- Keeping the patient's valuables safe.

The admitting department may be responsible for maintaining an organized and fair waiting system for arriving patients. Staff should be alert to situations that call for immediate medical attention or special handling. Most nonemergency patients can wait their turn, but anyone obviously suffering from physical or emotional stress should be given preference.

Admitting is usually responsible for providing patients with directions to service areas, such as

**Figure 5A.  Standardized Insurance Notification and Claim Form**
Developed by the Chicago Hospital Council.
NOTE: Copies of this multiple-copy form are forwarded to the group policyholder and insurance claim office. If payment is not received within a reasonable time, tracer copies are sent as a means of follow-up. If payment still is not forthcoming, a copy is sent to the advisory council of the Chicago Hospital Council's Chicago Area Hospital Admission Program for ultimate resolution of the claim.

*Chicago Area Hospital Admission Program*     **HOSPITAL INSURANCE CLAIM INQUIRY**

Date of Report

**1**

| Patient Name (Last) | (First) | (Init.) | Patient No. | Sex & Age | Date & Time Admitted |
|---|---|---|---|---|---|

Name & Address of Insured (Last, First, Init.)    S.S. No. of Insured    Relationship to Pt.    Date & Time Discharged

Phone No. of Insured    Occupation    Previous Admission Past 6 mos.   Yes ☐   Where?

**2** Name & Address of Group Policy Holder     Group Policy No.     Phone No.

Name of Insurance Co.     Empl. Clock or Badge No.

**3**    OTHER GROUP HOSPITAL COVERAGE?    Yes ☐   No ☐   Unknown ☐   **(IF 'YES' THIS SECTION MUST BE COMPLETED)**

Person Insured   (Last)    (First)    (Init.)    Employee Clock or Badge No.    Soc. Sec. No.    Blue Cross Group and Subscriber No. or Name of Commercial Insurer

Employer Name    Group Policy No.    Phone No.

**4**    **Name and address of Ins. Co. Claim Office.**     Hospital (Name & Address)

Eligibility Confirmed By:    Date    Benefits Quoted By:    Phone ☐   Ins. Form ☐

# T R A C E R

**INSTRUCTIONS TO HOSPITAL:**

    A.   FILL IN ADDRESS OF INSURANCE CO. CLAIM OFFICE AND ELIGIBILITY CONFIRMATION (NO. 4)—ABOVE.
    B.   COMPLETE SECTION I OF THIS FORM IN TRIPLICATE.
    C.   SEND PINK (PT. 2) COPY TO INSURANCE CO. CLAIM OFFICE. KEEP TWO COPIES INTACT FOR INTERNAL RECORDS.
    D.   IF ACCOUNT NOT PAID 15 DAYS AFTER FILING FIRST TRACER (INQUIRY) FILL IN SECTION II (BELOW) AND DISTRIBUTE AS OUTLINED.

**S E C T I O N I**

Give reason for Filing Inquiry (Check One)

| The Hospital Bill remains unpaid more than ☐ days after hospital billing date. | Amount Paid not in accordance with ☐ benefits originally quoted. | Other Reason(s) ☐ (Explain below) |
|---|---|---|

If more space needed, use back of form

Amount billed to Insurance Co.   $    Date    Amount Paid by Insurance Co. $

Hospital Representative

Inquiry form completed and submitted by:     Date

**S E C T I O N II**

If Inquiry (I) is NOT cleared within 15 days AFTER filing, fill in this section of the remaining copies and forward white copy to:

    THE ADVISORY COUNCIL OF THE CHICAGO AREA HOSPITAL ADMISSION PROGRAM, C/O OF THE CHICAGO HOSPITAL COUNCIL,
    840 N. LAKE SHORE DRIVE - SUITE 603, CHICAGO, ILLINOIS 60611

Check One:    Amount unpaid ☐ as of    Other problem ☐ unsettled as of    Response to initial inquiry ☐ unsatisfactory (Explain below)

If more space needed, use back of form

Second Section (copy) of Inquiry form completed & submitted by:    Name    Title    Date

CAHAP (75)-3

**ADVISORY COUNCIL**

Figure 5B.   Standardized Insurance Notification and Claim Form
(Tracer Copy)

laboratory and radiology, and for escorting them to the room. Patients requiring assistance with ambulation must be escorted at all times. Various personnel may escort the patients: hospital employees functioning as escorts, messengers, or transporters; volunteers; or admitting staff members.

A patient's valuables (money, jewelry, important documents) should be itemized on an envelope that also shows the patient's name and identifying data. The patient or his responsible representative should sign the envelope, as should the admitting staff member. The envelope should be sealed in the patient's presence and a receipt given to him. Last, the envelope should be deposited in a safe or other secure place. It is also advisable to record in a log all the valuables itemized on the envelope and the date they were received.

## Patient Information

Accurate and complete information on patients is essential to the efficient provision of health care. The information must be obtained tactfully and must be maintained in an organized, easily retrievable fashion. A system of individual folders containing all the documents and information acquired about each pending or newly admitted patient facilitates information storage and retrieval.

The major information items to be obtained for the patient register are:
- Admission date and time
- Patient's name
- Room and bed number
- Admitting physician
- Clinical service
- Admission type: emergency, urgent, elective
- Admission number

The patient register may be the means used to assign patient admission numbers if a unit numbering system is not being utilized. Numbers are assigned sequentially; the next available number is used for each new admission.

The American Hospital Association recommends that Social Security numbers *not* be used as the patient's admission or hospital identification number. The reasons for this recommendation are documented in AHA's statement *Against Use of Social Security Numbers for Hospital Medical Records,* which appears in appendix D. However, this recommendation does not preclude use of the Social Security number for other identification purposes.

Frequently, the insurer requires this item as a part of the patient information. Under provisions of the Privacy Act of 1974, however, public hospitals may in some cases be prohibited from requiring disclosure of patients' Social Security numbers.

The register can also serve as a master patient index, reducing duplication of data collection in various departments.

Other useful sociological and demographic information about patients includes:
- Address and phone number
- Sex and birth date
- Nearest relative or person to notify in case of emergency
- Employer's name, address, and telephone number
- Marital status
- Religion, church, and clergyman
- Race

Recognizing the need for uniform data collection, a group of health care organizations sponsored the development of the Uniform Hospital Discharge Data Set (UHDDS) in 1969. UHDDS specifies the minimum amount of data hospitals should collect on each patient. The majority of this information can be obtained upon admission. The American Hospital Association endorses and encourages the use of the data set in its statement *Health Data Systems,* which appears in appendix E.

## Financial Information

The financial and insurance information obtained is:
- Patient's financial coverage: Blue Cross/Blue Shield, Medicare, Medicaid, other government payments, commercial insurance, Workmen's Compensation, self-paying, charity, prepaid group program, or other
- Insurance policy or identification numbers
- Social Security number of patient and/or guarantor
- Verification of benefits (primarily for commercial insurer and Workmen's Compensation)
- Patient or guarantor's signature on payment guarantee, depending on who is ultimately responsible for payment of the bill if insurance coverage is not adequate
- Patient's signature allowing release of medical record information for insurance purposes

- Patient's signature assigning to the hospital insurance benefits not to exceed the amount of the hospital bill
- Receipts for deposits, if required

If the patient wishes a more expensive room accommodation than his insurance coverage allows, the admitting staff member should so inform him during the admitting interview, so that he is aware of his financial responsibility and can plan accordingly. Admitting should therefore have an up-to-date list of room charges on hand.

The American Hospital Association has developed a universal billing form, UB-16 (1976), for use with all types of health insurance coverage and all third-party payers (see figure 6, pages 30 and 31). The admitting department may be responsible for obtaining portions of the information required and the necessary signatures.

### Medical Information

The following medical information is obtained:

- Principal and secondary admitting diagnoses, and possibly the diagnostic codes (Many hospitals now use ICDA standard diagnostic codes to provide uniform information and clarity.)
- Patient's signature on treatment consents (usually just the general consent, but sometimes special consents as well)
- Attending physician's and/or surgeon's names and license numbers
- Previous admission dates, if any
- Patient's signature on releases and waivers, such as discharge against medical advice, refusal of treatment, leave of absence

### Patient Information Procedures

Much, if not all, of the sociological, demographic, financial, insurance, and medical information can be consolidated into one multipart admitting form containing appropriate information for each department requiring information about incoming patients. Figure 7, page 32, shows such a form.

It is important that the patient be accorded the opportunity to read and understand all the documents that he signs. This will aid in demonstrating the hospital's fulfillment of its responsibility in the event of future litigation. Furthermore, the patient has the right to be aware of and understand all procedures and transactions involving him, as indicated in the AHA's *A Patient's Bill of Rights* in appendix B.

When the patient admission interview has been completed and all required signatures have been obtained, the admitting staff member should make the patient's identification bracelet and imprinting plate from the information obtained during the interview. Generally, the following information is included on the bracelet and the plate:

- Patient's name
- Attending physician's name
- Room and bed number
- Admission number
- Admission date

Before the patient has left the interview area, the admitting clerk should review the patient's records for completeness and accuracy. After the patient has left, the clerk should distribute all the necessary documents to the various departments as required and insert the remaining documents in the patient's folder.

The folders can be stored in the admitting department's inhouse patient file in alphabetical order by patients' names. However, many hospitals prefer to keep these folders with the cashier. When a patient is ready for discharge, the cashier can easily review his financial status and determine whether financial arrangements or patient payment is necessary.

### Medical Staff Roster

Admitting may be responsible for maintaining the medical staff roster. The roster should indicate each physician's admitting privilege status (active, associate, courtesy) and whether privileges are currently in effect. If admitting privileges have been suspended, that fact should be noted. The roster should also list those physicians who have emergency or temporary privileges. It may be appropriate to list such physician's license number, which is sometimes required admitting information. Care must be taken to maintain the security and confidentiality of the roster.

### Directories

Admitting should maintain current lists of all outside organizations and parties with which it frequently deals. Examples are:

- Ambulance and taxicab companies
- Welfare agencies
- Nearby hospitals and other types of health care facilities
- Funeral homes

NOTICE: ANYONE WHO MISREPRESENTS OR FALSIFIES ESSENTIAL INFORMATION REQUESTED BY THIS FORM MAY UPON CONVICTION BE SUBJECT TO FINE AND IMPRISONMENT UNDER FEDERAL LAW

(1)

(2) HOSPITAL NO.　(3) PROVIDER NO.　(4) FED. I.D. NO.　(5)

(6) PATIENT'S LAST NAME　FIRST NAME　INITIAL　(7) STREET ADDRESS　CITY　STATE　ZIP

(8) PATIENT CONTROL NO.　(9) S-R　(10) BIRTHDATE　(11) ATTENDING PHYSICIAN　(12) ADMISSION-START OF CARE DATE　HR.　(13) QUALIFYING STAY DATES FROM　THRU　(14) H.H. PLAN EST.

(15) PRIMARY PAYOR - NAME　(16) INSURED'S NAME & RELATIONSHIP TO PATIENT　(17) CLAIM-CERTIFICATE - I.D. NO. (H.I.C.)　(18) GROUP NAME - NO.　(19) Y-N BENEFITS ASSIGNED

(20) SECONDARY PAYORS - NAMES　(21) INSURED'S NAME & RELATIONSHIP TO PATIENT　(22) CLAIM-CERTIFICATE - I.D. NO. (H.I.C.)　(23) GROUP NAME - NO.　(24) Y-N

(25)　(26)　(27)　(28)　(29) Y-N

(31)

(30) BILL TO

(32) TYPE OF BILL

PROFESSIONAL COMPONENTS
(33) RADIOLOGY　(34) PATHOLOGY　(35) OTHER　(36) MOST COMMON SEMI-PVT. RATE　(37)

| (38) CODE | (39) DESCRIPTION | (40) | (41) TOTAL CHARGES | (42) PRIMARY PAYOR | (43) SEC. PAYOR-ITEM 20 | (44) SEC. PAYOR-ITEM 25 | (45) PATIENT |
|---|---|---|---|---|---|---|---|
| TOTALS → | | (46) | (47) | (48) | (49) | (50) | (51) |

BLOOD RECORD (PINTS)　(52) FURN.　(53) REPLACED　(54) NOT REPLACED　(55) DED　(56) CHG/PT.　(57) BLOOD DED.　(58) INPATIENT DEDUCTIBLE　(59) DEDUCTIBLES　(60) DEDUCTIBLES　(61) DEDUCTIBLES　(62) PAID BY PATIENT

(63) STATEMENT COVERS PERIOD FROM　THRU　(64) P S CODE　(65) DIS HR　(66) COINSURANCE DAYS　(67) RATE　(68) L R DAYS USED　(69) COINSURANCE　(70) COINSURANCE　(71) COINSURANCE　AMOUNT DUE ▼

OCCURRENCES (72) DATE　(73) CODE　DATE AND CODE (74) DATE　(75) CODE　(76) COV DAYS　(77) N COV DAYS　(78)　(79) DUE FROM PRIMARY PAYOR　(80) DUE FROM SEC PAYOR ITEM 20　(81) DUE FROM SEC PAYOR ITEM 25　(82) DUE FROM PATIENT

(83) CODE　(84) PRINCIPAL DIAGNOSIS / NATURE OF ILLNESS　OTHER DIAGNOSES　(85)　(86) CODE　(87) CODE　(88) CODE　(89) CODE

(90) CODE　(91) DATE MO. DAY　(92) PRINCIPAL SURGICAL OR OBSTETRICAL PROCEDURE　OTHER PROCEDURES　(93)　(94) CODE　(95) MO. DAY　(96) CODE　(97) MO. DAY

(98)

(99)

(100) P I.P　(101) EMP. REL.　(102) REMARKS:　(103) I CERTIFY THAT THE CERTIFICATIONS ON THE REVERSE APPLY TO THIS BILL AND ARE MADE A PART HEREOF: PROVIDER REPRESENTATIVE X　(104) DATE

(105) VERIFIED NON-COV STAY DATES FROM　THRU　(106) PAYMENT DISTRIBUTION PROVIDER　PATIENT

(107) VERIFIED PATIENT LIABILITY BLOOD　CASH DEDUCT　COINSURANCE　(108) NON PYMT CODE　(109) DAYS USED

(110) R I　(111) ADJ CODE　(112) AMOUNT REIMBURSED　(113) DATE RECEIVED　(114) APPROVED BY (INITIALS)　(115) DATE APPROVED

UB 16-1976

Figure 6A. Uniform Billing Form, 1976 (front)
This form was developed by an American Hospital Association advisory panel.

SPACE FOR ADDITIONAL BILLING REQUIREMENTS AS NEEDED

Certifications Relevant to the Bill and Information Shown on the Face Hereof: Signatures on the face hereof incorporate the following certifications or verifications where pertinent to this bill:

1. If third party sponsor benefits are indicated as being assigned, on the face hereof; appropriate assignments by the insured and signature of patient or parent or legal guardian covering authorization to release information are on file. The hospital agrees to save harmless, indemnify and defend any insurer who makes payment in reliance upon this certification, from and against any claim to the insurance proceeds based in whole or in part upon an assertion that no valid assignment of the benefits to the hospital was made.

2. If patient occupied a private room for medical necessity, any required certifications are on file.

3. Physician's certifications and recertifications, if required by contract regulations, are on file.

4. For Christian Science Sanitoriums, verifications and if necessary, reverification of the patient's need for sanitorium services are on file.

5. Signature of patient or his representative on certifications, authorization to release information, and payment request, as required by Federal regulations and, if required by other contract regulations, is on file.

6. This claim, to the best of my knowledge, is correct and complete and is in conformance with the Civil Rights Act of 1964 as amended. Records adequately disclosing services will be maintained, and necessary information will be furnished to a governmental agency upon request.

7. For Medicare purposes: If the patient has indicated that other Health Insurance or State Medical Assistance Agencies will pay part of his medical expenses, and he wants information about this claim released to them upon their request, necessary authorization is on file.

8. For Medicaid purposes: I understand that endorsement hereon or deposit to the account of the within named payee is done with the understanding that payment will be from Federal and State funds and that any false claims, statements, or documents, or concealment of a material fact, may be prosecuted under applicable Federal or State laws.

ESTIMATED CONTRACT BENEFITS

Figure 6B. Uniform Billing Form, 1976 (back)

| | | | | | | |
|---|---|---|---|---|---|---|
| PATIENT NAME - LAST | | FIRST | | MIDDLE INITIAL | PHONE NO. | |

HENROTIN HOSPITAL
111 West Oak Street
Chicago, Illinois 60610

ADMISSION
SUMMARY
SHEET

MEDICAL RECORDS

BUSINESS OFFICE

**HENROTIN HOSPITAL** • 111 West Oak Street • Chicago, Illinois 60610       ADMITTING

Figure 7. Example of Admitting Form
Reprinted with permission of Henrotin Hospital, Chicago.
NOTE: Copies of the top one-third of this multiple-copy form go to the medical record department, reception desk, cashier, utilization review committee, and food service department. Copies of the bottom two-thirds go to the business office, data processing, credit manager, and physician(s). A copy of the entire form, excluding the guarantor and insurance sections, becomes the medical record face sheet, the top one-third of which is returned to admitting upon the patient's discharge.

- Public health agencies
- Mental health agencies
- Drug-abuse and alcohol-abuse programs
- Coroners
- Police and fire departments
- Local companies that provide group insurance

## Statistical Reports

If the hospital does not generate a computerized daily census and occupancy rate figures, it is usually the responsibility of admitting to compile such records manually from daily data on admissions, discharges, and transfers. If the hospital does have an automated census, it is admitting's responsibility to provide the input. In either case, the admitting staff must ensure that the required information is collected, maintained, and distributed in a timely, accurate, and organized fashion.

Admitting may also be responsible for providing input for various other patient statistical reports, such as those generated by medical records and data processing. Reports giving admitting information according to diagnosis, average length of stay, clinical service, patient classification, admitting physician, and surgical procedure are examples. Distribution of these reports to administration and outside organizations, such as hospital associations, boards of health, the Department of Health, Education, and Welfare, and the Joint Commission on Accreditation of Hospitals, may also be admitting's responsibility.

## Management Reports

Hospital administration and admitting management may wish to be apprised of admitting operations through a variety of management reports. Such reports are frequently composed of statistical data produced within the department. Examples of key operating figures that may be included are man-hours per admission, total cost per admission, and ratio of preadmissions to total admissions. These data can serve as basic performance indicators for the department. If data are compiled over a period of time, historical comparisons can be made of current versus past performance. Also, it may be possible to project future operations by using this information as a base. Figure 8, page 34, is an example of an admitting management report form.

## Bed Index

Admitting is responsible for maintaining an accurate and current bed occupancy index. Beds assigned to new patients should be designated in the index. Beds allocated to pending admissions also should be designated, but in a different manner from beds for inhouse patients.

Admitting must be kept apprised of discharges as they occur, so that a continual summary of bed availability can be maintained. A pending discharge system facilitates projection of upcoming available beds that can be tentatively assigned to pending admissions.

Various types of manual, mechanical, and computerized bed control systems and devices are described in chapter 6.

## Emergency Admissions

Emergency admissions are not scheduled and therefore create a problem in controlling beds. Although it is not possible to predict the daily bed demand for emergency admissions, reasonable estimates for the days of the week and the seasons can be projected by analyzing historical data. On the basis of such data, a specific number of beds can be reserved for potential daily emergency admissions. Many hospitals have found such a technique to be the most satisfactory solution to this ever-present problem. Although not perfect, it does present an objective approach.

Adequate procedures must be established for handling emergency admissions. Such admissions may be generated from the emergency department, doctors' offices, or outpatient clinics. If the clerical personnel in these various areas are not under the supervision of the admitting manager, adequate coordination and communication must be maintained between these areas and admitting to ensure that emergency patients are promptly admitted to the appropriate accommodation and that all necessary and available information is obtained.

The information requirements for emergency admissions are generally the same as for elective and urgent admissions. However, if the required information is not available at the time of admission, arrangements must be made for its collection at a later time. In such instances a bedside admission must be conducted or contact must be made with the patient's family to complete the information collection process. If the clerical staff in the originating area is not familiar with admitting procedures, it may be necessary for an admitting

## ADMITTING PERFORMANCE INDICATORS

| Period no. | DATES From | DATES To | 1 Total admissions | 2 Total nonemergency admissions | 3 Total department man-hours | 4 Total department dollars | 5 Total preadmitted patients | 6 Man-hours per admission | 7 Dollars per admission | 8 Preadmission ratio |
|---|---|---|---|---|---|---|---|---|---|---|
| 1 | | | | | | | | | | |
| 2 | | | | | | | | | | |
| 3 | | | | | | | | | | |
| 4 | | | | | | | | | | |
| 5 | | | | | | | | | | |
| 6 | | | | | | | | | | |
| 7 | | | | | | | | | | |
| 8 | | | | | | | | | | |
| 9 | | | | | | | | | | |
| 10 | | | | | | | | | | |
| 11 | | | | | | | | | | |
| 12 | | | | | | | | | | |
| 13 | | | | | | | | | | |
| 14 | | | | | | | | | | |
| 15 | | | | | | | | | | |
| 16 | | | | | | | | | | |
| 17 | | | | | | | | | | |
| 18 | | | | | | | | | | |
| 19 | | | | | | | | | | |
| 20 | | | | | | | | | | |
| 21 | | | | | | | | | | |
| 22 | | | | | | | | | | |
| 23 | | | | | | | | | | |
| 24 | | | | | | | | | | |
| 25 | | | | | | | | | | |
| 26 | | | | | | | | | | |

Column 1: From daily admission book
Column 2: From daily admission book
Column 3: From departmental personnel budget report
Column 4: From departmental budget report

Column 5: From daily admission book
Column 6: Divide column 3 by column 1
Column 7: Divide column 4 by column 1
Column 8: Divide column 5 by column 2

Figure 8. Example of Admitting Management Report Form
This form was developed by the Chicago Hospital Council's Hospital Central Services
Corp./Management Services Program.

staff member to go to that department to complete the admitting process, particularly if the patient is unable to come to the admitting department because of medical disability.

## Transfers and Referrals

Room transfers are arranged at the request of the patient, the physician, or the hospital.

If occupancy is high at the time of admission, the hospital may not be able to assign patients the type of accommodation they desire and therefore transfers them at a later date, when suitable accommodations become available. Other transfers that result from patients' requests occur when patients are advised that the probable length of stay will be longer than anticipated; requests for less expensive accommodations are frequently made.

The hospital transfers patients out of specialized nursing units when the treatment they require changes. The hospital may also initiate a request for a transfer when it is necessitated by other medical conditions, such as an infectious disease, irrational behavior, or a terminal illness. This transfer is usually from a semiprivate to a private room and is made upon the recommendation of the attending physician or the nursing service administrator.

If it becomes necessary to transfer patients in order to reallocate beds during high-occupancy situations or for other administrative reasons, the approval of the attending physician should be obtained.

The admitting department may be involved in transfers to other institutions. Coordination with the nursing department, the attending physician, the social service department, and other appropriate parties is required. The admitting department should not undertake the transfer of a patient to another facility without proper authorization from the appropriate individuals.

## Discharges and Deaths

The admitting department is frequently involved in the administrative aspects of discharging patients and also in arranging for patients who died in the hospital. The following considerations are important in ensuring the well-being of the patients and their families, maintaining the efficient operation of the admitting and related departments, and providing compliance with statutory and regulatory requirements.

When a patient is being discharged, the admitting department should be notified by the nurses' unit immediately, so that the bed index can be kept current. As previously discussed, a pending discharge system facilitates provision of information on projected bed availability in advance of actual discharge.

Close liaison should be maintained between admitting and the cashier to ensure that the patient has made suitable arrangements for the payment of financial obligations at the time of or prior to discharge. If the patient's financial folder is stored in the admitting department, it should be forwarded to the cashier or the business office for processing. Admitting may be responsible for notifying the other departments involved in the patient's discharge.

The admitting department may play a role in administering a discharge planning program by assisting with identification and recording of discharge planning needs at the time of admission. Admitting data may be used in assessing patients' long-term needs and prescribing treatment. Admitting staff may also assist with arrangements for transferring patients to suitable facilities at the time of discharge.

Discharge planning is a centralized, coordinated program that has been developed by an institution to ensure that each patient has a planned program for needed continuing care and follow-up. Discharge planning is essential to a concurrent patient care review system, whether conducted as part of utilization review or PSRO review. It ensures smooth transfer of a patient to another level of care once there is no longer a need for an acute care bed. Patient stays can be unnecessarily extended if discharge planning is delayed until the expected day of discharge. Payment for these "unnecessary" days may be denied under federal programs.

Upon the death of a patient, the admitting department usually handles the entire procedure, except for notifying the relatives, securing the autopsy permit, and completing the medical section of the death certificate.

The primary tasks to be accomplished are:

• Ensuring that the attending physician has notified the family of the death before the admitting department contacts the family. (The attending physician has the primary responsibility for notifying the family.)

- Ascertaining from the attending physician whether an autopsy is to be performed. If an autopsy is required or desired, it is recommended that the admitting department not be responsible for obtaining the autopsy consent. The attending physician should secure the consent because he is acquainted with the patient and the family and is in a better position to explain the medical reasons for the request. Admitting staff members are at a disadvantage in trying to persuade relatives to sign an autopsy consent, because their contacts with the patient and the family may be limited to admission.

- Notifying, as necessary, the coroner's office, police department, board of health, and other outside agencies. (See "Communication and Notification" later in this chapter.) Notification is made in accordance with local laws and regulations.

- Securing the nearest relative's signature on a release-of-remains authorization.

- Recording and surrendering the deceased's personal effects to the responsible representative, and obtaining the representative's signature upon the transfer of all recorded items.

- Completing the appropriate portions of the death certificate. Ensuring that the attending physician completes the medical portion and signs the certificate.

- Determining the family's preference regarding selection of a funeral home.

- Notifying the funeral home of when, in accordance with legal and autopsy requirements, the body may be taken. Obtaining the funeral home representative's authorization for the body, and arranging for the representative's access to the morgue. Providing the funeral home with a copy of the death certificate.

In conducting these affairs, the admitting staff must exercise the utmost discretion, tact, and sympathy in dealing with the patient's family. This is a time when a staff member's diplomacy and ability to make sound judgments are of vital importance.

In most hospitals, a person dead on arrival is not assigned a hospital number and admitted. A staff physician should not sign a death certificate unless the person was a previous patient for whom he was the last doctor in attendance. In such instances, where the cause of death can be satisfac-

torily stated, the admitting staff should assist the staff physician in completing the death certificate.

If none of the staff physicians was the deceased's last attending physician, the deceased's family should be referred to his previous doctor. The coroner's office should be notified in the event that the deceased's family indicates that the patient has not recently been seen by any doctor. In such instances, death certificates may be issued by that office.

## Inhouse Notification

The importance of adequate internal and external communication cannot be overemphasized. Various hospital departments and outside agencies and parties have a need to be informed of admitting department data and events.

The many departments that directly or indirectly serve patients should be notified of all admissions, discharges, and transfers so that their services can be directed to the appropriate patient and location. (Various communication and information system alternatives are discussed in chapter 6.) The following should usually be notified, either by admitting or another department, depending on the type of communication and information system used in the hospital:

- Laboratory (if preadmission or admission testing is required)
- Radiology (if preadmission or admission testing is required)
- Food service
- Switchboard
- Information or reception desk
- Utilization review coordinator
- Chaplain
- Medical records
- Attending physician, and also consulting physician and/or surgeon
- House staff
- Business office
- Nurses' station
- Escort service
- Data processing
- Volunteers
- Pharmacy
- Cashier
- Housekeeping
- Social services

Frequently the admitting department is the hub of this notification system. If this system is not functioning properly, the entire patient care system of the hospital can be jeopardized.

## Reporting Cases Required by Law

Admitting is frequently responsible for reporting various cases, described below, to appropriate authorities: the police, the coroner, or the department of health. Local and state laws governing the reporting of various types of cases to these three offices vary. When information is provided to various municipal or state departments, the date, time, and person notified, as well as the name of the person notifying the department, should be shown on the report form.

The conditions requiring reporting should be discussed with the proper officials in the area. Generally, the following types of cases are reported:

- To the police department: patients dead on arrival when death resulted from other than natural causes, cases that in any respect give evidence of being criminal in nature, traffic accident injuries, gunshot wounds, poisonings, dog bites, drownings, suicides and attempted suicides, child abuse, drug overdoses.
- To the medical examiner's and/or coroner's office: patients dead on arrival; deaths occurring without previous medical attention, as defined by state statute; homicides; suicides; deaths caused by a communicable disease; deaths due to accidents on the job; any sudden deaths arousing suspicion of crime or foul play; manslaughter cases, whatever the cause; criminal abortions; accidents causing death directly or indirectly as a result of gunshot wounds, poisonings, and burns and scalds due to fires, explosions, and conflagrations; deaths occurring under the influence of an anesthetic, whether in an operating room or in a patient's room; drownings; deaths caused by acute alcoholism or drug addiction; deaths occurring in the hospital as a result of injury sustained there.
- To the department of health: The department of health should be notified about all cases in which it has a particular interest. A list of the types of cases requiring reporting can be obtained from the appropriate city or state agency and should be incorporated in the admitting department policies and procedures manual.

The hospital should keep a complete and accurate file on all such cases.

## Inquiries on Patients' Conditions

If the hospital does not have an information desk, the admitting department may be responsible for reporting patients' conditions. The department should not volunteer information beyond that specifically authorized for release to inquirers. Condition reports, which are sent to the admitting department from nurses' units at stated times during the day, should be sufficiently complete so that the usual questions asked by relatives and friends can be answered readily and accurately.

Admitting may also be responsible for notifying a designated clergyman of a patient's medical condition or death.

# References

American Hospital Association. *Discharge Planning for Hospitals.* Chicago: AHA, 1974.

_____. *Hospital Medical Records: Guidelines for Their Use and the Release of Medical Information.* Chicago: AHA, 1972, pp. 61-64.

_____. *Medical Record Departments in Hospitals: Guide to Organization.* Chicago: AHA, 1972, pp. 11-18, 67-79.

_____. *Postmortem Procedures.* Chicago: AHA, 1970, pp. 17-54.

American Medical Record Association. *Glossary of Hospital Terms.* Chicago: AMRA, 1974, pp. 8-10, 18-20, 62.

American Medical Record Association and Greater Portland Admitting Officers Association. *Management Guide for Admitting Personnel.* Chicago: AMRA, 1975, pp. 27-66.

Hospital Research and Educational Trust. *Guide for the Utilization Review Coordinator in a Quality Assurance Program.* Chicago: HRET, 1974.

Seawell, L. V. *Hospital Accounting and Financial Management.* Berwyn, IL: Physicians' Record Co., 1964, pp. 169-84.

*Uniform Hospital Abstract; Minimum Basic Data Set: A Report of the United States National Committee on Vital and Health Statistics.* Chicago: Hospital Research and Educational Trust, 1973.

United Hospital Fund of New York; Training, Research, and Special Studies Division. *The Admitting System: A Special Study in Hospital Systems and Procedures.* New York City: the Fund, 1965.

chapter *4*
# *Legal Considerations*

Some of the legal matters that arise in the day-to-day activities of the admitting department are described briefly in this chapter. This discussion is only a summary and does not encompass all of the legal aspects of admitting problems. Furthermore, because laws vary from state to state, local legal counsel should always be consulted.

The admitting manager should read at least one comprehensive reference on hospital law. Pertinent texts are listed at the end of this chapter.

## RECORDS AS LEGAL DOCUMENTS

Many hospital records are initiated in the admitting department, and it is essential that these records be accurate and complete. Because the admitting manager cannot possibly foresee which of these many records may sometime be used in litigation, he should emphasize the legal implications of every entry when training admitting personnel. He should also point out that any omission or mistake on a record can undermine confidence in the record as a whole; doubt may arise as to whether other information has been reported and accurately recorded.

Although most admitting documents are maintained with the patient's financial or medical record, the admitting department may find it necessary to maintain a master patient index of all admissions and discharges. This index, and any other records, should be retained in accordance with requirements specified in federal, state, and local statutes and administrative rules and regulations and in conformance with the hospital's operating needs.

## POLICIES AND PROCEDURES MANUAL

Admitting department procedures should be evaluated to determine whether they conform to applicable standards of practice. All admitting policies approved by the governing board and all procedures should be in writing as the department's policies and procedures manual. In the event the hospital's admitting practices are questioned, the manual governing the actions of the admitting staff serves to show the hospital's adherence to applicable standards of good practice.

All admitting department procedures should be followed exactly as outlined in the manual. If the admitting manager believes that a procedure can be improved, his suggested modification should be approved by administration before it is put into effect. Approval is especially necessary if the proposed change affects the reporting of cases to outside agencies. Failure to comply with regulations of the medical examiner, coroner's office, board of health, or police department may be a violation of the law (see "Reporting Cases Required by Law" in chapter 3).

## CONSENTS FOR TREATMENT AND SPECIFIC PROCEDURES

It is standard practice to secure a general consent from each patient authorizing all treatment and tests regarded by the attending physician as necessary. Special consents for specific procedures such as surgery, anesthesia, and radiological therapy are advised. Generally, a consent should be obtained for all procedures requiring a specific explanation to the patient (see page 9). Figures 1, 2, and 3 on pages 10, 11, and 13 contain examples of general and special consent forms.

Admitting personnel should explain the general consent form to incoming patients; the explanation should be simple and nontechnical. The attending physician generally is responsible for obtaining special consents, and this is done at the time he explains the special procedure to the patient. The patient or his legal representative not only should consent to but also should understand the treatment, tests, or procedures.

A consent for each surgical procedure should be obtained in writing, to avoid misunderstandings about the nature and extent of the operation to be performed. The consent form should also authorize the administration of any anesthetic and the performance of any operations that the surgeons in attendance deem advisable. Many forms also state: "If it is necessary to amputate or remove any material, the hospital or its agents are authorized to make proper disposition thereof." If an amputation or removal is anticipated, the consent should state that fact in writing and name the part involved.

Obtaining the consent to operate on minors, particularly those in their late teens, may present a problem. Generally, the consent of a parent or guardian is necessary for an operation on a minor, except in an emergency. Even then, it is sound practice to obtain parental consent as soon as possible. The fact that a person is under the legal age, which varies from state to state, does not make him incapable of giving his consent. However, it is safer to also secure the approval of the parents.

Some state statutes expressly provide that a minor may consent in his own behalf to alcohol or drug treatment, to the treatment of venereal disease, and to the performance of an abortion. Such statutes may prohibit notifying or securing the permission of parents or guardians. In this area particularly, hospital legal counsel should be consulted.

Minors who may give consent that is recognized legally (in more than drug, venereal disease treatment, and abortion situations) are known as emancipated minors. Such minors are allowed to keep their own earnings and are not subject to parental control. If a minor is living away from home and earning his own living, generally he may give his consent because he is responsible for himself. A married woman under the age of majority generally does not need her parents' consent for an operation. Neither, generally, is her husband's consent required. Local legal counsel should be consulted as to applicable state law.

In obtaining consent for minors, it is generally safest to secure permission from the parents or guardians (unless, as with drug, alcohol, and venereal disease treatment, abortions, and sterilizations, this is prohibited by state law). If the parents are not available, an older brother or sister of legal age may not legally consent unless he or she is appointed legal guardian of the minor. If the parents are living apart, the wisest policy is to secure the consent of both, although practical difficulties may present themselves, so that the consent of one parent with established legal rights to custody may have to suffice.

Parents who refuse to agree to an operation on a minor, even when death may ensue without it, are within their rights. They should, however, be asked to sign a written refusal absolving the hospital, physician, and hospital personnel from failure to provide the medically recommended treatment. Parental authority can be overruled only by court appointment of a guardian to replace the parents and give the necessary legal consent (see appendix C).

## CONSENTS FOR EMERGENCY OPERATION AND TREATMENT

If an emergency patient enters the hospital in a condition in which he is unable to sign a consent form (for example, an unconscious state) or if he cannot understand it, an attempt should be made to obtain consent from another responsible party. Whenever possible, situations of this type should be referred to administration for approval.

If consent cannot be obtained and serious impairment or death will result from nontreatment, the physician may administer the necessary treatment. When a patient is fully conscious, consent should be obtained even though the physician is authorized to perform emergency treatment. An unconscious patient requiring immediate treatment is an emergency patient who may receive treatment without consent.

## RELEASE FROM RESPONSIBILITY FOR ANESTHESIA AND TRANSFUSIONS

Consent to a surgical procedure does not automatically imply consent to the administration of anesthesia. Therefore, formal consent should be obtained for the use of anesthetics. The consent form for surgery may specify the use of an anesthetic, so that a patient has to sign only one form rather than two. A signed release such as this will not, of course, absolve the hospital from liability for any injury resulting from negligence for which it is institutionally responsible. Generally, however, such a release disproves any allegations of assault and battery, the legal term applied to procedures performed without consent.

Most hospitals do not secure signed releases from blood donors. Because donors are fully conscious and have an understanding of the process, their cooperation may be considered as implied consent to the performance of the procedure. However, consideration should be given to obtaining consent from the recipient of a blood transfusion. Transfusions can be covered in the general consent form.

## DISCHARGES AGAINST MEDICAL ADVICE OR FOR DISCIPLINARY REASONS

A release from responsibility should be obtained whenever a patient is determined to leave the hospital against the advice of his attending physician and the administration. This signed form does not release the institution or the physician from liability for any negligence or malpractice that may have resulted in harm to the patient while hospitalized; however, it clearly suggests that whatever happens after the patient leaves the hospital is not the result of the institution's failure to render care, but, instead, the unwillingness of the patient to accept the care available to him. This signed form is evidence to disprove any accusations that the hospital refused care to the patient or discharged or forcibly removed him prematurely.

Whether or not a patient may be discharged for disciplinary reasons depends on his condition and the severity of the breach of discipline. The fact that he does not obey the rules may not be sufficient justification for removing him from the hospital. The difficult patient may be discharged from the hospital under the following circumstances: (1) his removal from the hospital will not jeopardize his well-being, and/or (2) his presence in the hospital is a menace to the recovery and health of other patients.

## ABORTIONS, MISCARRIAGES, AND STERILIZATIONS

Patients entering a hospital for an abortion, miscarriage, or sterilization introduce special legal problems that may affect admitting and treatment procedures. Virtually all hospitals, nonsectarian and religious, have different rules for such cases. State laws also vary greatly. Specific guidance should be obtained from local legal counsel.

## AUTOPSY

### Consents

Although it should never be the responsibility of the admitting staff to secure an autopsy permit, staff should understand the legal implications of such permits and the requirements of state laws. There is no uniformity among states with respect to such laws, so the following general guidelines may not apply in every state.

Every consent for autopsy should be in writing. The form should provide space for the signatures of the person consenting and of two witnesses. In general, consent for an autopsy should be given by the person normally entitled to possession of the body for disposition. Ordinarily, this right rests with the surviving spouse. Sons and daughters generally come next, if they are of age. All competent offspring have an equal legal voice in this decision; the law does not make the oldest son or daughter the representative of the other offspring.

In the absence of any special disposition by a will, a surviving spouse married to the patient at the time of death usually has the right to possession of the body for disposition, which is paramount to the rights of the next of kin. In the event that the surviving spouse was separated from the patient at the time of death or refuses to exercise the right of disposition, a waiver of that right may be implied. The right may therefore inure to other relatives. However, if the spouse promptly asserts the right to possession of the body for disposition, this right must be recognized. The effect of a divorce is to terminate the legal relationship between spouses; upon the death of one, the other has no right of disposition over the spouse's body.

In the absence of a living spouse, there is generally recognized to be an equal right among surviving adult offspring to give consent for an autopsy, provided none have alienated themselves from the deceased. Any one adult son or daughter may provide the consent.

When no surviving parent, spouse, or adult offspring exists, minors of sufficient maturity who are the next of kin are sometimes recognized to have the right to consent to autopsy on a parent. In the absence of a living spouse, adult offspring, or minors of sufficient maturity, parents may give the consent.

Whenever there is more than one member of a group, such as children of the deceased, authorized to give consent to autopsy, most states require the consent of only one member. Very few states address the situation when one member of the group gives consent but another refuses consent to an autopsy. The hospital's legal counsel should be consulted, and guidelines established for handling such situations in accordance with state law.

Executors of wills and administrators of estates, as distinguished from the family, have no right to the dead body for disposition. The fact that the administrator must pay the funeral expenses does not make him the authorized custodian of the body.

By the same token, he has no authority to consent to autopsy.

If, in the absence of next of kin, a close friend is given possession of the body for disposition, he or she then has authority to consent to autopsy.

**Restrictions**

The individual who has authority to permit an autopsy also has the right to restrict it. Any limitations on the authorization must be observed, unless a full autopsy has been ordered by the public health official empowered to do so, such as the medical examiner, when the circumstances of death are such that state law compels an examination.

To avoid any misunderstanding, the extent of the autopsy should be explained when the authorization is obtained. A consent authorizing examination to ascertain the cause of death impliedly permits the removal of organs necessary for microscopic examination, provided no tissue is retained. Therefore, it is important that the autopsy consent specifically include a provision permitting the retention of diseased tissue or organs.

The law of most states provides that no postmortem examination may be made of a deceased patient having no known relatives until a diligent effort has been made to locate any next of kin or close friends. This rule is obviated if the case belongs to the medical examiner's or coroner's office; medical examiners' cases or coroners' cases may preclude the hospital pathologist from carrying out some postmortem examinations.

Hospitals may be further restricted by state statutes that specify the time period within which an autopsy must be performed.

## RESPONSIBILITY FOR PAYMENT

It is important for the admitting department to ascertain not only who is responsible for payment of the hospital bill but also who is financially able and willing to pay. The age of the patient may be significant in this respect. In general, if a minor resides with his parents and they provide the major portion of his financial support, they can be held responsible for his hospital or medical services. For services rendered to an emancipated minor, the parents are not liable unless they give consent for those services and agree to pay. A person under legal age may make a binding agreement to pay a hospital bill, but may not have the ability to pay it. It is advisable in such instances to ask a responsible adult to guarantee payment.

A minor is usually not responsible for an adult patient's hospital bill, even though he may sign a guarantee of payment. Any son or daughter who is an adult or emancipated minor under state law may guarantee payment of a parent's hospital bill. In addition, any responsible adult can serve as guarantor of a patient's hospital bill if he has signed an agreement to this effect.

A guarantee of payment is valuable only if the person signing it actually is able to meet the payments. The admitting department usually has the responsibility during the admitting interview to establish the guarantor's probable ability to pay. If this information is not obtainable, the patient should be referred to the credit manager.

In the case of a married woman, the husband ordinarily is responsible for payment of his wife's bill. The woman, by express agreement in writing, may make herself solely responsible. Although a husband is legally bound to support his wife and family, this obligation does not prevent a wife from obtaining necessities for the family on her own responsibility and personally agreeing to pay for them. In some states, her contract is not binding unless she has property of her own.

When a husband is separated from his wife because she left him without cause, he generally is relieved of the responsibility to pay her bill. Divorce also terminates the obligation of the husband to support his former spouse, except to the extent provided by agreement as to the award of any alimony.

A wife is not usually responsible for the support of her husband, but some states have statutorily recognized the liability of a wife for her husband's medical expenses on the basis that they constitute a necessary family expense. The adoption of the Equal Rights Amendment would materially affect payment responsibility; husband and wife would be equally responsible for the payment of all debts.

Brothers and sisters requesting treatment for siblings are under no obligation to pay unless they are adults and have signed an agreement to act as guarantors.

## LIENS

Many states have hospital lien statutes that create a lien in favor of the hospital without the necessity of the consent of the patient. Such a lien is an obligation imposed by law upon the person responsible for the injuries for which a patient is being treated or upon that person's insurance carrier. Money is paid to the hospital out of the fund due to the patient in settlement or by judgment. Blank lien forms usually can be obtained from the county clerk's office and are returned to the same office upon completion for proper filing of record there.

Hospitals in states without hospital lien statutes are unable to secure advance liens unless patients are willing to authorize them voluntarily.

## WORKMEN'S COMPENSATION

Workmen's Compensation laws provide standard benefits for work-related sicknesses or accidents. A list of these benefits should be available in the admitting department for reference. The admitting manager may deem it advisable to routinely phone patients' employers to determine whether standard benefits are available or whether there are limitations that will affect the benefits.

## VALUABLES
### Safekeeping of Patients' Property

Admitting personnel should urge every patient to send valuables home or to check them in the safe. Patients should be informed, either by admitting personnel or a patient information booklet, that the hospital is not liable for the loss of or damage to property that is not surrendered for safekeeping. A patient who insists on storing valuables in his room should be asked to sign a form releasing the hospital from liability.

Despite these disclaimers, the hospital still may be responsible for loss through carelessness. When a patient surrenders valuables for safekeeping, a contract is made with the hospital that the property is to be returned upon demand or discharge. This contract does not release the hospital from responsibility for negligence. The hospital is expected to exercise reasonable prudence to protect these valuables.

Possession of patients' property by the hospital includes the responsibility to protect it in the interests of the patient. When property in the custody of the hospital is demanded under legal process by a third party, the institution must ensure that the proceedings are valid before surrendering any valuables. However, the hospital is not required to litigate the dispute for the patient.

### Releasing Valuables of Deceased Patients

The hospital should not turn over the property of a deceased patient to anyone except the legal representative of the estate. When a patient dies leaving a will, the person named therein as the estate's representative is the executor. The executor, upon filing the will for probate, obtains certificates evidencing appointment, which are often referred to as letters testimentary. They are then entitled to receive the deceased's property for distribution in accordance with his will.

When a patient dies leaving no will, the next of kin may petition the court to be appointed administrator. The person named by the patient upon admission as the nearest relative is not necessarily the one to receive the property of the deceased. If the hospital releases valuables of a deceased patient to someone other than the appointed administrator or executor, it actually may be performing an unauthorized act. Therefore, admitting personnel should insist on seeing court-certified evidence of the executor's or administrator's appointment before surrendering valuables. The hospital may also wish to obtain a receipt for the property transferred to the representative.

If there is no next of kin and the decedent has left no valid will, the hospital should release the deceased's property to the public administrator of the county in which the patient last resided. The public administrator pays the obligations of the estate in the order of their priority, investigates and collects other prospective assets such as bank accounts, and attempts to locate relatives.

If the patient, upon admission, signs an agreement depositing with the hospital money to be applied periodically for payment of the bill, only that left on deposit upon the patient's death becomes the property of the estate.

## RESTRICTIONS ON ADMISSIONS

Any hospital that offers emergency service may be prohibited from refusing that service to a true emergency patient in need of immediate medical attention.

With the foregoing exception, however, admission need not be granted to all who apply. Although public hospitals are licensed to accept and are therefore obligated to accept all patients living within their service area who seek admission, private hospitals are not so obligated. Refusal to admit a patient must not, however, be based on the applicant's race, color, religion, or national origin.

Nonemergency patients may validly be refused admission to an acute general hospital under the following circumstances:

- If hospital care is not considered medically necessary, as determined by a staff physician.
- If occupancy levels are high and some persons seeking admission have less pressing ailments.
- If accommodations are full.
- If the patient refuses to pay the regular rates when believed to be financially able to do so.
- If the patient is suffering from a chronic condition.
- If the patient needs only convalescent care.
- If the hospital does not have the appropriate facilities for treating the patient. For instance, special hospitals (such as psychiatric, chronic disease, rehabilitation, and tuberculosis institutions) are licensed to treat patients with special medical problems and, because they are equipped to treat only such patients, do not admit those with different treatment needs.

Policies and procedures should be in effect for referring or discussing all questionable cases with appropriate medical and administrative staff. Depending on the particular situation, patients denied admission should be referred to the hospital's outpatient department or to another health care facility or community agency, or otherwise assisted in some way.

## PRIVILEGED COMMUNICATION

Medical records and all information obtained by a physician from his patient are confidential. This information should not be disclosed by admitting personnel to unauthorized individuals without the express written consent of the patient or the person who legally represents him.

It is customary for a patient to disclose all pertinent information about his malady to enable his physician to diagnose and treat the condition. Sometimes this information is so personal that if it were to be publicly circulated it would prove both embarrassing and detrimental to the patient. In recognition of this situation, a privileged communication statute has been enacted in many states. Under such a statute, medical information is inadmissible as evidence in all legal cases in which this right has not been waived, except when a court has ordered that such information be admitted in evidence.

A privileged communication statute recognizes the fact that a patient may be somewhat handicapped in his relationship with a physician. The patient often is suffering from pain or weakness, ignorant of the nature or extent of his injury or illness, driven by necessity to call for professional assistance, and obliged to submit to the intimate disclosure involved in physical examination. As such, he occupies a dependent position in relation to his physician. The statute is therefore intended to encourage full and frank personal disclosures of physical conditions by relieving all patients, regardless of financial status or physical state, from fear of any embarrassing consequences of such disclosures.

## INFORMATION FOR LAWYERS, INSURANCE COMPANIES, OR OTHERS

No medical information should be given by admitting personnel to a lawyer, an insurance company, or any party other than the patient, until hospital authorities are satisfied that the patient has authorized the requested disclosure.

## WILLS

As a general rule, hospital employees should not participate in the preparation or witnessing of a patient's will. Patients should be advised to obtain the services of a lawyer to draw up the will. Witnesses should be secured from among their friends or relatives rather than from hospital personnel.

# References

American Hospital Association. *Hospital Medical Records: Guidelines for Their Use and the Release of Medical Information.* Chicago: AHA, 1972, pp. 4-9, 14-20.

_____. *Postmortem Procedures.* Chicago: AHA, 1970, pp. 17-54.

American Medical Association. *Medicolegal Forms with Legal Analysis.* Chicago: AMA, 1973.

California Hospital Association. *Consent Manual.* 8th ed. Sacramento, CA: CHA, 1970.

Cheifetz, W. *Consent Manual.* Phoenix: Arizona Hospital Association, 1971.

Colorado Hospital Association. *Consent Manual.* Denver: CHA, no date.

Epstein, R., and Wolf, N. *Manual of Consent Forms.* Albany, NY: Hospital Association of New York State, 1974.

Hayt, E. *Law of Hospital, Physician and Patient.* 3rd ed. Berwyn, IL: Physicians' Record Co., 1972, pp. 83-158, 419-512, 573-88, 1023-150.

New Jersey Hospital Association. *Consent Manual.* Princeton, NJ: NJHA, 1972.

New Mexico Hospital Association. *Legal Handbook.* Albuquerque, NM: NMHA, 1972.

North Dakota Hospital Association. *Consent Manual.* Grand Forks, ND: NDHA, 1972.

Texas Hospital Association. *Hospital Legal and Consent Manual.* Austin, TX: THA, 1963/1964-.

University of Pittsburgh, Health Law Center. *Hospital Law Manual.* 2nd ed. Administrators' vols. 1 and 1A. Germantown, MD: Aspen Systems Corp., 1974, Admitting and Discharge sections 1-4, Governing Board section 5, Financial Management sections 1 and 8-10, Medical Staff sections 1-3.

Washington State Hospital Association. *Consent Manual.* Seattle: WSHA, 1972.

Wisconsin Hospital Association. *Consent Manual.* rev. ed. Milwaukee: WHA, 1969.

_chapter_ **5**
# Physical Characteristics

When a hospital is building a new admitting department or evaluating an existing one, consideration should be given to the department's location, decor, and work areas and how these all contribute to the efficient and effective performance of tasks and procedures.

## LOCATION

Among the many factors that influence the location of the admitting department are its accessibility to incoming patients, the location of the departments with which admitting works most closely, the volume of admissions, the hospital's communications system, and the hospital's credit policy.

Because the admitting department's chief function is the reception and admission of patients, it should be easily accessible to and on the same level as the main entrances of the building. Incoming patients and the persons accompanying them are under emotional tension and may be easily confused if the admitting department is not designated clearly. Therefore, an identifying sign should be close enough to the main entrance to be readily seen.

Because of the numerous people—patients, visitors, hospital personnel, and medical staff—who use the admitting department's services, the department should be centrally located and in proximity to the main lobby. The lobby provides a place where companions may comfortably wait while patients are being admitted. Public telephones and rest rooms should be provided. Also, patients should be able to reach the interviewing area easily when summoned.

When main lobbies are continually being used at or near full capacity, the noise level may be distracting and available seating at a minimum. In such situations, a separate waiting area for incoming patients and their companions should be considered.

The physical condition of many incoming patients necessitates that the admitting department be located near elevators. This is particularly important for cardiac and obstetrical patients, who require immediate care, often in areas of the hospital most quickly reached by elevators.

Whenever possible, the admitting department should be located near those departments with which it has considerable interaction, in order to facilitate the prompt handling of patients and other related duties. Admitting should be located within easy access of the following: cashier, medical records, reception/information desk, switchboard, patient accounts, business office, laboratory and radiology, and social service.

In the interest of operating efficiency, the admitting department should be located close to the medical record department if a unit numbering system is in use. Each time a patient is admitted, the master patient index has to be checked to determine whether a previous record exists. If a record does already exist, it is sent to the admitting department for coordination with the patient's admission and for reuse of the original record number. If a patient is being admitted for the first time, the medical record department provides a number.

Depending on the financial policies of the hospital, it may be advantageous to locate the admitting department near the financial department. Incoming patients with financial and credit problems are usually referred to the patient accounts manager so that matters can be resolved in private. Patients may be referred to the cashier if they must pay an advance deposit or wish to turn over valuables for safekeeping.

Admitting should be conveniently accessible to primary laboratory and radiology facilities. Separate laboratory and x-ray functions within the admitting department are becoming increasingly popular; they can facilitate the admission process by enabling preadmission and admission tests to be administered immediately at the point of entry rather than in several areas throughout the hospital. Such an approach may be considered by hospitals with a well-established preadmission program or those with a large volume of patients requiring a standard admission test series.

## FURNISHINGS AND DECOR

Because first impressions are lasting impressions, it is important that a patient's initial contact with a hospital be a favorable one. An attractively furnished admitting department contributes enormously to creating a favorable first impression.

Above all, a stereotyped institutional appearance should be avoided. The atmosphere of the admitting department should be light and cheery. It should give the impression of comfort and, at the same time, inspire confidence. To achieve this, the walls should be papered attractively or painted in warm, relaxing colors. Upholstered furniture should be colorful but not gaudy. The atmosphere can be enhanced by hanging colorful paintings on the walls and carpeting the area. All furnishings should conform to the requirements of the Life Safety Code.

Since one of the objectives in furnishing the admitting department is to make it as unofficelike as possible, all forms and supplies should be stored in furniture that blends with the surroundings. Often, it is better to keep only a limited amount of supplies in the office. A larger inventory can be stored in an adjacent room or area.

During an admitting interview, patients often divulge information of a confidential nature. Therefore, it is advisable to provide several private offices or cubicles for interviewing purposes. The offices should be large enough to accommodate a desk and chair for the admitting staff member and sufficient chairs for the patient and others who may accompany him.

## FUNCTIONAL AREAS

The amount of space required for the admitting department obviously varies, depending on the number of daily admissions. Each hospital must determine its own needs and plan its admitting department to best meet them.

Sample layouts for admitting departments in hospitals of 100 and 500 beds are shown in figures 9 and 10, pages 49 and 50. The examples are for illustrative purposes only; they are not intended to depict the ultimate admitting department layout.

A brief description of each functional area within the typical admitting department follows.

### Waiting Area

A waiting area serves as a lounge for incoming patients and their companions. It should be functionally suited to their physical and psychological needs. Public telephones and rest rooms should be nearby. The waiting area should also be convenient to the admitting interview offices and other areas to which patients may be referred before the admitting process is completed.

# CENTRAL ADMITTING DEPARTMENT WITH ADJACENT MEDICAL RECORD DEPARTMENT FOR A 100-BED HOSPITAL

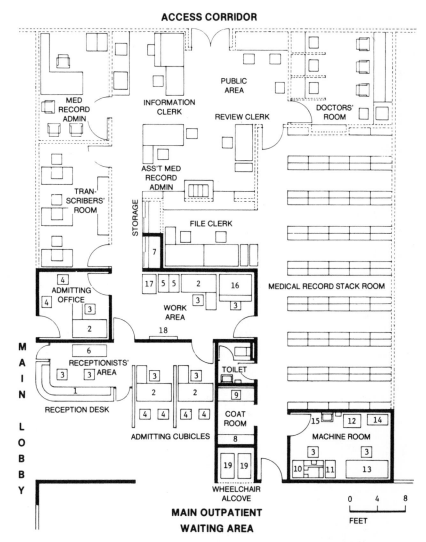

PARTITIONS SHOWN WITH DOTTED LINES INDICATE MEDICAL RECORD DEPARTMENT AREAS

NOTE:  COAT ROOM AND TOILET ALSO SERVE MEDICAL RECORD PERSONNEL

## L E G E N D

| | | |
|---|---|---|
| 1. Control counter | 9. Sink top cabinet unit | 15. Wall-hung lavatory |
| 2. Clerical desk | 10. Manual plate printer | 16. Master patient index |
| 3. Secretarial swivel chair |     (keyboard controlled) |     (elevator file) |
| 4. Straight chair | 11. Plate file cabinet | 17. Appointment index |
| 5. File cabinet | 12. Electrostatic copier |     (mobile, visible type) |
| 6. Utility table | 13. Work table with knee- | 18. Current bed occupancy |
| 7. Built in supply closet |     hole and base cabinets |     index (insert type) |
| 8. Shelf and hanger rail | 14. Supply cabinet | 19. Admittance chair |

Figure 9. Example of Layout of Central Admitting Department with Adjacent Medical Record Department in a 100-Bed Hospital

Reprinted from *Administrative Services and Facilities for Hospitals: A Planning Guide,* published by the U.S. Government Printing Office.

NOTE: Partitions shown with dotted lines indicate medical record department **areas.** Coat room and toilet also serve medical record personnel.

# CENTRAL ADMITTING DEPARTMENT WITH ADJACENT MEDICAL RECORD DEPARTMENT FOR A 500-BED HOSPITAL

(Generally similar for a 300-bed hospital except fewer admitting offices and/or cubicles may be indicated.)

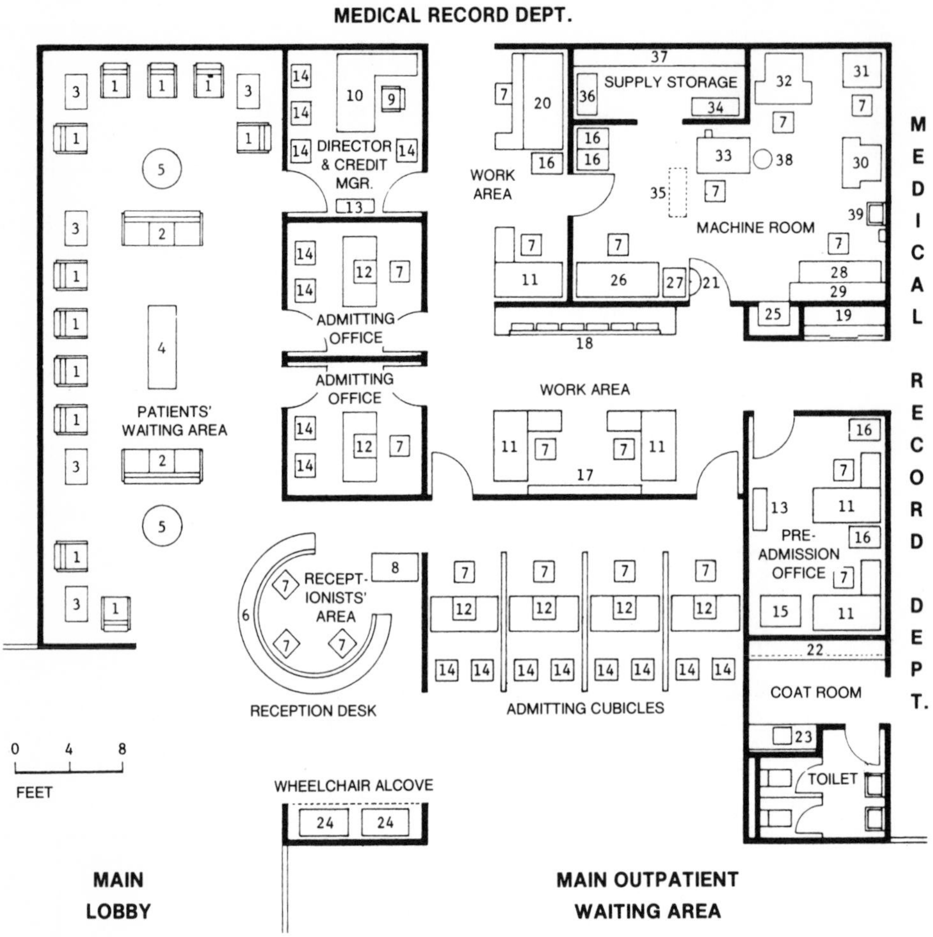

Figure 10. Example of Layout of Central Admitting Department with Adjacent Medical Record Department in a 500-Bed Hospital (Generally similar for a 300-bed hospital, except that there might be fewer admitting offices and/or cubicles.)

NOTE:   COAT ROOM AND TOILET ALSO SERVE MEDICAL RECORD PERSONNEL.

## LEGEND

1. Lounge chair
2. Three place sofa
2. Lamp table
4. Center table
5. Health literature display table
6. Control counter
7. Secretarial swivel chair
8. Utility table
9. Management swivel chair
10. Management desk
11. Clerical desk
12. Teletypewriter desk
13. Bookcase
14. Straight chair
15. Appointment index (mobile, visible type)
16. File cabinet
17. Current bed occupancy index (insert type)
18. Bed availability registers (illuminated signal type)
19. Built in supply cabinet
20. Master patient index file (elevator type)
21. Pass window in door with hinged shelf
22. Shelf and coat hanger rail
23. Sink top cabinet unit
24. Admittance chair
25. Universal air tube station
26. Work table with kneehole and base cabinets
27. Plate file cabinet
28. Work table
29. Shelf over work table for remote tape punches
30. Automatic plate printer (punched tape controlled)
31. Manual plate printer (keyboard controlled)
32. Electrostatic copier
33. Imprinter with lister (foot controlled)
34. Shelf truck
35. Shelf truck work position
36. Supply cabinet
37. Shelving for notification form stock
38. Trash receptacle
39. Wall-hung lavatory

Reprinted from *Administrative Services and Facilities for Hospitals: A Planning Guide,* published by the U.S. Government Printing Office.

NOTE: Coat room and toilet also serve medical record personnel.

In a hospital where the daily volume of scheduled admissions is small and multiuse waiting areas such as the lounge area of the main lobby are convenient to the admitting interview offices and other referral areas, a separate waiting area for incoming patients may not be necessary. Seating equal to one-third of the average daily number of inpatient admissions should be available.

## Reception Desk

The admitting department's reception desk is manned by one or more clerks, who receive patients, record their arrival, and assign them to interviewing offices.

## Interviewing Offices

Interviewing offices or cubicles serve as work areas in which admitting staff can interview patients privately to obtain comprehensive sociological, demographic, and financial information for records. Because cubicles afford less privacy than offices, they may be less satisfactory for admissions. When the patient's history has been obtained in advance of his arrival and all that remains to complete the admission is to obtain his signature on one or two forms or give him some routine instructions, an admitting cubicle is adequate.

Interviewing offices should be well-lit, well-ventilated, and soundproof.

## Work Area

The work area can perhaps be considered the hub of the admitting department, in that much of the routine clerical work associated with the admission, transfer, and discharge of patients is carried on here. The area should provide sufficient space for the personnel and equipment necessary to carry out such functions as maintaining various directories, reports, and records; and checking, issuing, and filing forms and notices.

## Preadmission Office

This area provides space for one or more clerks, who gather preadmission information and handle bed assignments. Separate laboratory and x-ray facilities for preadmission testing may or may not be part of this office.

## Machine Room

This room usually contains equipment used in preparing patient identification plates, cards, and bracelets and preparing and duplicating daily reports. Pending patient admission files and small supplies of forms may also be kept here.

Because the equipment produces a noise level that would be distracting to other areas of the department, it is usually totally enclosed, and sound-absorbing measures are taken to keep the noise level within acceptable limits.

A pass-through window from the machine room to the work area may be a worthwhile addition.

# Reference

U.S. Department of Health, Education, and Welfare; Health Care Facilities Service. *Administrative Services and Facilities for Hospitals: A Planning Guide.* Washington, DC: Government Printing Office, no date, pp. 12-25.

## chapter 6

# Equipment and Systems

With the increasing complexity of admitting activities, many time-saving and labor-saving devices have been developed for the purpose of facilitating admitting routines. It should be noted, however, that the most sophisticated equipment and materials are not necessarily the most appropriate solution to a problem. For example, a computerized system may not be what is needed in a disorganized department that has manual admitting procedures. Suitable manual systems and procedures must be operating before more sophisticated methods can be effectively introduced.

The cost for new equipment should be justified. Simply because a new device can save several hours of staff time each day does not mean that the labor savings will offset the acquisition, operating, and maintenance costs of the equipment. Manual systems are completely adequate to meet the needs of many admitting departments. The actual needs and capabilities of the department should be assessed before a decision is made to install new equipment or upgrade existing equipment.

When the merits of various systems are being evaluated, the following questions should be asked:

- What advantages has automated equipment over manual operations?
- How much space in the admitting office can be allotted to equipment?
- Will the equipment under consideration materially reduce the length of time required to admit patients?
- Is the equipment or system under consideration capable of accommodating increases in work volume, and, if so, to what degree?
- What is the initial cost of the equipment? The estimated annual upkeep?
- What savings can be effected by utilizing the equipment for purposes in addition to admitting department needs?
- How much special training is required to enable personnel to operate the equipment?

- Is the equipment compatible with other equipment, the allotted space, and other physical characteristics of the department?
- Are special forms and supplies required and readily available?

In this chapter, equipment and systems are classified according to the admitting department function they are intended to facilitate: data collection, duplication, communication and data transmission, and management of bed resources. The terms *manual, mechanical,* and *computerized* designate relative levels of sophistication.

## DATA COLLECTION

The ever increasing information needs of health care have meant an increase in the data collection responsibilities of the admitting department. Consequently, many new devices as well as modifications of older methods have been developed for this purpose.

### Forms

The basic information collection and storage media used in most admitting departments are forms. The best designed forms are those that facilitate the recording of all necessary information in the simplest possible manner.

Administrators and admitting managers should be alert to all ways and means of simplifying and standardizing information collection. Standardized forms facilitate the work of hospital employees and make comparison possible with the same types of information from other sources.

When suitable standard forms are not available, the admitting department should design its own. The questions asked of patients, various notification responsibilities, policies and procedures— these and other factors determine the content and format of each form. In addition, all information should be sequenced in a logical, easily understandable fashion. A printer with experience in the specialized area of forms design should be used when a department chooses to devise its own forms.

Forms should be reviewed periodically to ensure the relevance and currency of the types of information requested. Information needs should be carefully evaluated so that only necessary items are included. All items that have proved unessential should be eliminated.

Many admitting procedures are accomplished through the use of multiple-copy snapout forms.

One type utilizes carbon paper; the other is treated with a pressure-sensitive coating for duplication of the original copy. When the form has been completed, the various copies are separated and distributed as required. See figure 7, page 32, for an example of an admitting form.

Each hospital, with the assistance of legal counsel, should design its release and consent forms so that they are kept to a manageable number and apply to all or most needs. Such a practice will reduce confusion about which form is appropriate for which occasion and will reduce the number of signatures required of the patient or his legal representative. See figures 1, 2, and 3, pages 10, 11, and 13, for examples of consent forms.

### Admission Numbers

Admission numbers can be assigned by use of a patient register, as described earlier on page 28. Numbers are assigned sequentially, by using the next available number for each new admission. This is frequently the simplest method available. However, such a system is readily subject to human error: transcription errors can occur, duplicate number assignments are possible, and numbers can be skipped. If this method is selected, care must be taken to train personnel properly and review all work output. Failure to do so can result in sizable charge and billing errors in the business office as the result of misassigned numbers.

Various types of mechanical devices, such as number generators and stamping machines, are available that preprint numbers on admitting forms, labels, and patient folders. Such an approach reduces transcription and duplication errors. A disadvantage is that supplies of preprinted materials must be carefully controlled if the integrity of the numbering system is to be maintained. If some unused materials are lost, gaps in the numbering system will result and may cause distortions in related systems that depend upon the admission number. For example, hospitals that assign admission numbers consecutively often use this system as a means of compiling daily patient volume figures. Problems can also arise in the coordination of preprinted forms with each other and with other documents relating to a patient with a particular number; the matching process can become difficult without properly functioning operating routines.

Computer-generated lists of unassigned admission numbers are frequently utilized in admitting departments. Although such computerized systems may not reduce initial transcription and duplication errors, they frequently incorporate a check digit in the admission number that automatically identifies misassigned numbers. If data processing facilities are readily available to the admitting department, such lists can be easily and inexpensively obtained. In addition, computerized admitting systems may automatically assign admission numbers.

The foregoing discussion does not consider manual, mechanical, or computerized unit numbering systems, which operate on the principle that the same identifying number is used each time a patient is readmitted. Such a system facilitates medical record identification and retrievability. However, care must be taken in patient number assignment and control. Close communication and coordination with the medical record department must be maintained. If control mechanisms fail, the improper assignment of numbers will result not only in billing errors but also in improper merging and location of medical records.

### Data Input

If a hospital does not use a computerized admitting system, all information gathering and storage must be done manually or mechanically via handwritten or typed documentation. If a hospital does use a computerized system, data can be entered by the following means: key-punch machine with punch cards, standard terminal with magnetic tapes or disks, or cathode ray tube (CRT) with direct on-line input. With the first two types of systems, information is typed and produced on punch cards, tapes, or disks, which are subsequently processed through a computer. With the CRT, information is entered in the computer at the same time it is being typed on the keyboard of a computer terminal.

The development of the CRT has enhanced computerized admitting systems. Many CRT admitting systems are commercially available. The great advantage of CRTs is that information can be directly and immediately entered into the system without the need for extensive training of personnel. Information is readily displayed on a screen similar to a television screen. Employee orientation to the proper use of a CRT can be conducted in a minimum amount of time; the skill required is not substantially more than that of a typist. The capacity of a computerized admitting system using a CRT is such that when a patient is admitted or preadmitted, all the information gathered on him, as described in chapter 3, can be entered via the CRT.

Accuracy, timeliness, and completeness of input must be stressed with any computerized system because the speed of processing compounds and magnifies errors if the input is incorrect or inadequate. Input discipline must be maintained. As previously emphasized, successful conversion to a computerized system depends upon properly functioning manual routines prior to automation. Automation alone will not correct or improve a poor system.

The advantages of a computerized system are many. Preadmission tests can be ordered. Deposits can be collected and recorded prior to admission. An admission number can be assigned. A patient master record can be initiated and stored permanently without detailed interviewing or processing on the day of admission. A current admission record is also produced. Patient charges are automatically entered without cumbersome requisition completion and distribution. File security is maintained through an identification/authorized access system incorporated into the computerized admitting system. Visual or automated edit verification of input before transmission is available to ensure the accuracy of all data entered into the system. This last aspect of a computerized admitting system is vital to efficient, effective operation and generation of high-quality output.

## DUPLICATION

Many departments within the hospital, as well as outside organizations, have a need for information obtained by the admitting staff. The multipart forms described on page 54 can in large measure fulfill these needs. Their use should be encouraged whenever many different parties must be provided with admitting information, inasmuch as the cost per copy is usually less than that of a mechanically duplicated copy.

However, in many situations it may not be practical to generate a separate copy of the multipart form for each party requiring information. For instance, information may be required on an exceptional basis only, or the functional need may not be compatible with the format of the form. The equipment and systems described here represent available alternatives and should be evaluated in light of the duplication needs of the department.

## Embossers and Imprinters

If embossers and imprinters are in use, the admitting staff selects the information necessary for the metal or plastic imprinting plate and produces the individualized plates by typing on the keyboard of an embosser. Usually embossed on the plate is such information as the patient's name, attending physician, date of admission, room and bed number, and admission number. Then the plate, whenever inserted in an imprinter, stamps the identifying information on requisitions and other documents.

Frequently, admitting must initiate preadmission or admission tests by using a plate and an imprinter. In addition, after a patient has been admitted, his plate is forwarded to the nurses' unit for continued use in imprinting service requisitions or other documents originating at that location. The plate is usually durable enough to allow for repeated imprinting before it becomes worn, thus providing standardized information that is imprinted clearly and neatly on all documents upon which it is used.

## Mimeograph and Liquid Duplicators

Although mimeograph and liquid duplicators have been available for many years and are somewhat outdated, they may adequately fulfill the duplicating needs of the small admitting department that does not have heavy duplication demands. These devices are inexpensive to operate, require little maintenance, and provide reasonably good copies if only a small volume is needed. However, duplication is time-consuming because it is first necessary to make a stencil in order to reproduce the desired copy. The duplication process itself is time-consuming and can be messy. If the admitting department has a need for high-quality copy in a minimum amount of time, other methods of duplication may be more appropriate and cost-effective.

## Photocopiers

Admitting departments are increasingly utilizing photocopiers as the demand placed upon the departments for information collection and dissemination grows. Although this equipment can be costly to acquire and operate, the speed of production and quality of copy frequently justify its use. There is no need to make a stencil of each item to be duplicated; the original document serves as the master copy.

There are two basic types of photocopiers: wet and dry. The wet copier uses a liquid as the printing medium, the dry uses a powder. Various types of paper may be required. Some photocopiers use plain bond, others use specially treated paper.

Sizable cost variances exist, depending on the equipment and supplies selected. Careful evaluation and consideration of the various types of equipment and related supplies available can reduce the expense involved.

Photocopy equipment can play an important role in helping the admitting department to meet the increasing information requirements of third-party financial reimbursers. Patient insurance identification cards frequently are reproduced with such equipment in order to create an exact copy of much of the information required for reimbursement purposes. Various reports and documents emanating from the admitting department can also be reproduced by photocopying.

## Electronic Printers

Most reports generated by a computer can be produced in quantity by an electronic printer. The advent of data processing has therefore reduced the report production and duplication responsibilities of many admitting departments. Many of the reports described in chapter 3 can be produced and duplicated by data processing equipment.

## COMMUNICATION AND DATA TRANSMISSION

Because so many different departments and parties within the hospital must be able to communicate with the admitting department, it is necessary to ensure that adequate systems are available for the timely and accurate transmission of information. All of the departments and parties listed on page 18 must be able to provide information to and/or receive information from admitting. Many alternatives exist for accomplishing this task.

## Messengers

A well-functioning, properly designed messenger service can expedite the flow of information not only between admitting and related departments, but throughout the hospital. This basic method of information transfer serves many hospitals well; large as well as small institutions have found it to be an effective method of interdepartmental communication. However, the labor costs involved can be sizable. An automated system in conjunction with a messenger service may be required in order to reduce or contain operating costs.

### Telephones

Although often taken for granted, the telephone is the most obvious automated communication mechanism used in the admitting department. Frequently, a simple telephone call can transmit the necessary information to meet operational requirements within a minimum amount of time. Many departments also use a telephone intercom system as part of their intra-office communication network. The telephone should be used whenever no suitable alternative method of communication exists in a hospital. The following automated communication systems, however, can reduce the time consumed by telephone calls.

### Pneumatic Tubes

With a pneumatic tube system, documents are placed in small receptacles that move to their destination by suction through pneumatic tubes. This system transports documents rapidly. Admitting departments frequently use such a system for communication with nurses' units, the business office, and other departments.

### Electronic Photocopy Transmitters

Electronic information transfer equipment operates in conjunction with photocopiers so that reproduced copy is transmitted electronically to a remote destination. Careful analysis and evaluation should be undertaken prior to obtaining such equipment. It is quite expensive, and the quality of copy received can vary. Transmission time is slow —one to four minutes. Maintenance requirements can be sizable. Despite these factors, some admitting departments, especially those in a large hospital complex, may have a genuine need for such a capability. If so, this equipment may provide a satisfactory data transmission solution.

### Remote Printers/Writers

Three of the most common remote printers/writers are teletype machines, electronic writers, and tele-autowriters. These various alternatives utilize either a keyboard or a handwriting instrument as the means of data entry.

All three options can facilitate the communication process for admitting and related departments. The configuration selected should be based on the abilities of the admitting staff and the needs of the department and hospital. Such equipment can be appropriate in large hospitals; small hospitals may have difficulty justifying the expense involved.

### Computers

Computer systems provide a fast, comprehensive means of data transmission. One of the primary features of a computerized admitting system is its ability to notify all concerned departments and parties of all admissions, discharges, and transfers. These notifications are made promptly and accurately, with a minimum of manual assistance. Likewise, departments having a need for specific admitting information are able to inquire via a computer terminal rather than slower, and frequently less accurate, traditional communication methods. Ancillary department orders and test results can also be transmitted via the terminal.

Financial data, such as charges, insurance information, and deposit status, can be communicated to the business office. In turn, the business office has immediate inquiry access to these data when required. Census and statistical data may also be accommodated in the system as an aid in medical record statistical compilations as well as in the utilization review process. Assignment of initial length-of-stay estimates and notification of patient review and insurance benefit cutoff dates can be performed.

## MANAGEMENT OF BED RESOURCES

Two of the primary responsibilities of the admitting department are the assignment of beds and maintenance of an accurate bed occupancy/availability summary. These tasks can be accomplished with the assistance of a variety of bed control devices.

### Manual Displays

The two basic manual configurations are bed control boards and bed card display racks. Both depend upon continual manual input and updating in order to remain current. Frequent telephone or messenger contact with the nurses' units must be maintained. Cards or markers are used to indicate bed status. Color-coding or symbols highlight key information on a patient, such as clinical service; sex; age; and status in terms of pending admission, admission, pending discharge, discharge, or transfer.

## Mechanical Displays

Mechanical displays are an elaboration of manual displays. Lights, rather than cards or markers, are used to indicate bed status. Different-colored lights signify different bed statuses: bed occupied, bed available, pending admission, discharge, and transfer.

The advantage of a mechanical over a manual system is that transmission of bed status information is expedited. Each nurses' unit has its own control panel, which is used to maintain the master bed control display in admitting. By means of switches or dials, the nursing staff provides admitting with the most current bed status information. The cashier, food service, pharmacy, and housekeeping may also have display/control panels, so that service needs can be promptly satisfied.

A disadvantage of the mechanical system is information inflexibility. Manual systems allow for a much greater variety of information display. The information displayed by a mechanical system is relatively fixed. Large hospitals may find that their bed-size capacity necessitates use of a mechanical system. Small hospitals can usually control beds adequately with a manual system. A key factor with both kinds of systems is training personnel to continually update the information maintained, so that an accurate bed summary is always available.

## Computerized Systems

A computerized admitting system has the ability to provide complete, current, and immediate bed availability/occupancy reports. Instantaneous information is available to all areas having terminal inquiry capability. Current bed reservation lists and patient waiting lists can also be maintained.

A well-designed, fully installed computerized admitting system is capable of assisting not only in management of bed resources, but also in data collection, duplication, and communication and data transmission, as discussed earlier in this chapter. However, such systems are highly sophisticated and expensive and require extensively trained personnel. They are suitable only for hospitals that can afford the necessary investment, require the potential level of performance, and employ personnel capable of properly understanding and operating the equipment. For many hospitals, manual or mechanical alternatives are a more practical approach.

## chapter 7

# Ambulatory Care Registration

For purposes of this chapter, ambulatory care includes both the emergency department and outpatient services that are operated as integral parts of the hospital.

The American Hospital Association has developed the following classifications of hospital ambulatory care patients:

- Emergency outpatient—a patient who is admitted to the emergency, accident, or equivalent service of the hospital for diagnosis and treatment of a condition that requires immediate medical, dental, or allied services.

- Clinic outpatient—an outpatient who is admitted to a clinical service of the hospital for diagnosis or treatment in a formally organized unit of a medical or surgical specialty or subspecialty. The clinical service involved assumes overall medical responsibility for the patient.

- Referred outpatient—an outpatient who is admitted to a special diagnostic or therapeutic service of the hospital. The referring physician assumes medical responsibility for the patient.

This chapter discusses registration of these patients and scheduling of their ambulatory care.

## POLICIES

In some hospitals the responsibility for ambulatory care registration is included within the admitting department or the organizational unit having responsibility for admitting. All patient admissions, whether inpatient or outpatient, are consolidated within one department. Whether admissions and registration are consolidated or separate, the hospital must make provision for admitting patients who come to the ambulatory care services and then require hospitalization. Policies need to be established on how to handle such situations. The internal workings and requirements of the hospital must also be considered in establishing ambulatory care services policy.

Many of the same policy considerations apply to the registration of ambulatory care patients as apply to the admission of inpatients. External as well as internal factors bear heavily on ambulatory care functions, just as they do on inpatient functions. Accreditation and professional standards must be maintained. Third-party reimbursement regulations must be met. Recognition of and adherence to legal requirements are necessary. Public relations are crucial, because a large number of patients are seen and because ambulatory care services are frequently regarded as a major element in meeting the health care needs of the community served.

Some policy factors that are specifically relevent to ambulatory care registration are as follows:

- The emergency department's classification, if a categorization of emergency services is used in the hospital's geographic area.

- Types of services offered and referral options.

- Charity services offered.

- Hours of operation.

- Information requirements.

- Patient community served.

- Organization and administrative responsibility.

- Staffing requirements.

- Reporting requirements and lines of communication.

- Financial and reimbursement requirements.

- Public relations and the image that the hospital wishes to project.

- Fee schedules and payment requirements.

- Confidentiality of information.

Policies on the above matters may differ substantially between the emergency department and outpatient services. In the development of policies, such matters must be considered within the operating context and intended objectives of the individual units and the hospital.

In short, all the factors more fully described in chapter 1 must be considered in the ambulatory care setting. Policies must be established that address these various factors. As with inpatient admitting, the development of a well-organized, comprehensive, and clearly written policy and procedure manual will assist in compliance with all policy matters.

## ORGANIZATION AND PERSONNEL

Although many hospitals now incorporate the ambulatory care registration and appointment functions within the admitting department, other hospitals include these functions within the ambulatory care, financial, medical record, nursing, or other related department. As with inpatient admissions, placing responsibility for information collection and appointment scheduling with medical or other personnel who have unrelated primary duties can reduce the accuracy and efficiency of the registration process. To ensure a properly functioning registration system, it is generally desirable to utilize clerical staff specifically trained in the duties and procedures of registration and scheduling. These personnel should be placed under the supervision of a person who fully understands and appreciates the importance of obtaining complete, accurate information and operating an effective appointment system. (A sample job description for an outpatient clinic coordinator, which delineates some registration supervision functions, is presented as appendix F.)

Adverse ramifications may result throughout the hospital if the ambulatory care registration staff is not qualified or properly trained. Incomplete, inaccurate, or irretrievable medical records may be compiled—a factor that could hinder the delivery of optimum patient care and compliance with accreditation standards. Necessary financial and insurance information may not be acquired—a factor that could impair billing and collection operations and impede cash flow. An improperly functioning appointment scheduling system may cause excessively long waiting times, poor utilization of professional personnel, missed appointments, and bad public relations.

An in-service training program can be developed that not only addresses the administrative aspects of patient registration but also trains clerical personnel in basic medical terminology and in the identification of emergency medical situations. Such medical training should not be intended to supplant professional treatment, but to alert professional staff to serious situations that might not otherwise be readily identified because of operating conditions.

Depending on the patient population served and difficulties involved in adequately meeting its needs, some ambulatory care services may wish to utilize special personnel for certain circumstances, such as interpreters and patient ombudsmen.

## FUNCTIONS AND PROCEDURES

The need for accurate, comprehensive information gathering is equally as important for ambulatory care registration as for inpatient admission. One of the major components of the registration clerk's duties is collecting patient financial, sociological, and demographic data. Frequently, some medical information is also recorded during this process. A uniform minimum basic data set for ambulatory care, similar to the uniform hospital discharge data set for inpatients, has been developed. Although this data set has not been universally adopted by the nation's hospitals, its contents are regarded as the minimum requirements for adequate ambulatory care registration.

The major items of information to be recorded by registration staff and medical personnel are as follows:

- Patient identification: full name, hospital identification number (serial or unit number).
- Residence: full address including zip code, telephone number.
- Date of birth.
- Sex.
- Financial coverage or expected sources of payment, including necessary identification numbers: Medicare, Medicaid, other government programs, Blue Cross/Blue Shield, commercial insurance, Workmen's Compensation, prepaid group program, self-paying, charity, or others.
- Provider (usually physician) identification: full name, identification number, professional address, profession or specialty.
- Date of encounter.
- Place of encounter: emergency department or outpatient service.
- Reason for encounter: principal problems, complaints, or symptoms in patient's words.
- Findings: history, examination, diagnostic test results.
- Diagnosis and/or problem.
- Services and procedures: diagnostic, therapeutic, preventive.
- Itemized charges, based on recorded services and procedures.
- Disposition: no follow-up planned; return, time specified; return, as necessary; telephone follow-up; referral to other provider; return to referring provider; admission to hospital; other.

Individual hospitals may wish to record supplementary data for particular purposes, such as billing and collection, utilization review, and statistical reporting. (Sample emergency department registration forms, figure 11, appear on pages 62 and 63.) In addition, the registration staff should be responsible for seeing that all necessary signatures of patients or other responsible parties are gathered for such items as consents, assignments of insurance benefits, and payment guarantees.

Registration staff frequently are responsible for collecting payments or for directing patients to the cashier. Some hospitals institute a cash collection system for those patients who do not have adequate insurance coverage. The relatively small dollar amounts of ambulatory care bills combined with the high cost of providing service may make such a practice necessary.

Consideration must be given to the best time for collection: should payments be made prior to or upon completion of service? Public relations matters, operating routines, and financial policy will determine which approach is most appropriate.

To ensure that fees are fair and equitable, a sliding scale or series of classifications might be developed for assessing the base charge. Such fees can be structured on the amount of time used in treating the patient, the degree of difficulty of the case, or the procedure performed.

Registration clerks may be responsible for charge accumulation and final recording. Initially, medical personnel may record the test, treatment, or supply item used. The clerk then records the appropriate charge for the items and determines the total amount owed. Automated charge input and accumulation systems along with associated forms have been developed to facilitate this process (see the "Equipment and Systems" section of this chapter).

Appointment scheduling may be another major function of the registration staff. A well-coordinated patient scheduling system can have a significant, beneficial impact on ambulatory care activities by reducing patient waiting time, improving utilization of physicians and nursing personnel, reducing congestion and improving traffic flow, improving public relations, and improving utilization of facilities.

**HENROTIN HOSPITAL** 111 WEST OAK STREET, CHICAGO, ILLINOIS  **EMERGENCY DEPT. 19517**

| DATE | TIME | PATIENT BROUGHT BY | FROM | | AMB. | STRCH. | WH. CH. | PATIENT NO. 3429989 |

| PATIENT'S NAME (LAST) | (FIRST) | (MIDDLE) | SEX | AGE | BIRTH | RACE | CIV. STAT | REL. |

| STREET ADDRESS | CITY | STATE | ZIP | PHONE NO. |

| NOTIFY IN EMERGENCY | RELATIONSHIP | PHONE NO. | BIRTH PLACE | FAMILY NOTIFIED |

| STREET ADDRESS | CITY | STATE | ZIP | ADM. ROOM | P.I.L. | C.P.D. NOTIFIED |

EMPLOYER (CHECK ONE) — EMPLOYED BY — PATIENT'S ☐ NEAREST REL. ☐ | OCCUPATION | ER PVT WC ☐☐☐ | ADM. M.D. NOTIFIED | TIME

| EMPLOYER'S ADDRESS | PHONE NO. | PT. SOC. SEC. NO. | AICDA CODE |

INSURANCE TYPES AND NUMBERS

**ADMITTING**

**NURSE**

NURSE'S SIGNATURE

CONDITION ON ARRIVAL AT E.R. — GOOD ☐ FAIR ☐ POOR ☐ SHOCK ☐ HEMORRAGE ☐ COMA ☐ | TEMP. | PULSE | RESP. | B.P. | ALLERGIES

PHYSICAL EXAM:

PROVISIONAL DIAGNOSIS:

TREATMENT ORDERS:

☐ TET. TOX.:
X-RAYS ORDERED:
LAB. TESTS ORDERED:
DRUGS:
SOLUTIONS:
OTHER:
REMARKS:

**PHYSICIANS REPORT**

☐ PVT. M.D. ☐ ON CALL M.D. | NOTIFIED ☐ YES ☐ NO | MESSAGE LEFT | TIME | PHYSICIAN:

DISPOSITION OF PATIENT — HOME ☐ BACK TO WORK ☐ OTHER ☐ | CONDITION OF PATIENT: | TIME DISCHARGED FROM E.R.

FOLLOW-UP INSTRUCTIONS: | I ACKNOWLEDGE RECEIPT OF WRITTEN FOLLOW-UP INSTRUCTIONS.

_____ PATIENT'S SIGNATURE

**AUTHORIZATION FOR EMERGENCY ROOM TREATMENT**

1. THE UNDERSIGNED HAS BEEN INFORMED OF THE EMERGENCY SERVICES CONSIDERED NECESSARY FOR TREATMENT, AND THAT THE TREATMENT AND PROCEDURES WILL BE PERFORMED BY PHYSICIANS, MEMBERS OF THE HOUSE STAFF AND EMPLOYEES OF THE HOSPITAL. AUTHORIZATION IS HEREBY GRANTED FOR SUCH TREATMENT AND PROCEDURES. THE UNDERSIGNED AGREES THAT NO GUARANTEE OR ASSURANCE HAS BEEN MADE AS TO THE RESULTS THAT MAY BE OBTAINED. I HAVE BEEN INFORMED AND UNDERSTAND THAT I MUST FOLLOW THE ABOVE PATIENT INSTRUCTIONS.
2. AUTHORIZATION IS HEREBY GIVEN TO RELEASE MEDICAL INFORMATION TO HEALTH CARE PROVIDERS IN CONNECTION WITH FURTHER TREATMENT WHICH MAY BE RENDERED AND FOR COMPLETION OF MY INSURANCE CLAIM. I UNDERSTAND THAT I AM FINANCIALLY RESPONSIBLE TO HENROTIN HOSPITAL FOR THE CHARGES MADE BY THEM FOR SERVICES RENDERED.

DATE _____ SIGNED X _____
PATIENT OR AUTHORIZED PERSON

**MEDICAL RECORDS**

Figure 11A. Example of Emergency Department Registration Form

Reprinted with the permission of Henrotin Hospital, Chicago.

NOTE: Copies of this multiple-copy form go to the medical record department, the clinic/doctor, and the business office.

**HENROTIN HOSPITAL** **111 WEST OAK STREET, CHICAGO, ILLINOIS** **EMERGENCY DEPT.** 19518

| DATE | | TIME | PATIENT BROUGHT BY | | FROM | | | | | AMB. STRCH. WH. CH. | | PATIENT NO. |
|---|---|---|---|---|---|---|---|---|---|---|---|---|

PATIENT NO. **3429970**

| PATIENT'S NAME (LAST) | (FIRST) | (MIDDLE) | SEX | AGE | BIRTH | RACE | CIV. STAT | REL. |
|---|---|---|---|---|---|---|---|---|

| STREET ADDRESS | CITY | STATE | ZIP | PHONE NO. |
|---|---|---|---|---|

| NOTIFY IN EMERGENCY | RELATIONSHIP | PHONE NO. | BIRTH PLACE | FAMILY NOTIFIED |
|---|---|---|---|---|

| STREET ADDRESS | CITY | STATE | ZIP | ADM. ROOM | P.I.L. | C.P.D. NOTIFIED |
|---|---|---|---|---|---|---|

| EMPLOYER (CHECK ONE) | EMPLOYED BY | OCCUPATION | ER PVT WC | ADM. M.D. NOTIFIED | TIME |
|---|---|---|---|---|---|

PATIENT'S ☐ NEAREST REL. ☐

| EMPLOYER'S ADDRESS | PHONE NO. | PT. SOC. SEC. NO. | AICDA CODE |
|---|---|---|---|

| INSURANCE TYPES AND NUMBERS | PAT.TYPE | HOSP. SERV. | DR'S NO. | FIN. CLASS | NO INS. |
|---|---|---|---|---|---|

PAT.TYPE **E** HOSP. SERV. **ER**

| DESCRIPTION | CODE 378 | X | CHG. | DESCRIPTION | CODE 378 | X | CHG. | DESCRIPTION | CODE 378 | X | CHG. |
|---|---|---|---|---|---|---|---|---|---|---|---|
| Emergency Room Fee | 1000-2 | | | **E.R. SUP. & EQUIP.** | | | | **PHYS. THER. EQUIP.** | | | |
| **PROCEDURE** | | | | Catheter Tray-Foley | 5000-4 | | | Cane - Adjustable | 4378000-0 | | |
| Aspiration | 2000-8 | | | Catheter Tray-French | 5001-2 | | | Crutches | 4378001-8 | | |
| Incision Drainage | 2001-6 | | | Cautery Disp. | 5002-1 | | | Rib Belt XL | 4378002-6 | | |
| Intubation | 2002-4 | | | ENT Tray w/Meds. Packing | 5003-9 | | | Rib Belt M & L | 4378003-4 | | |
| Debridment | 2003-2 | | | Suction | 5004-7 | | | Surgical Shoes | 4378004-2 | | |
| Removal Foreign Body | 2004-1 | | | Eye Tray & Serv Meds. | 5005-5 | | | Cervical Collar | 4378005-1 | | |
| Sutures | 2005-9 | | | Levine Tube | 5006-3 | | | **SPLINTS** | | | |
| Muscle Repair | 2006-7 | | | Oxygen | 4368000-5 | | | Finger Splint | 9000-6 | | |
| Gastric Lavage | 2007-5 | | | Steri Strips | 5007-1 | | | Leg Splint-Short | 9001-4 | | |
| Tendon Repair | 2008-3 | | | Venous Press. Set | 5008-0 | | | Leg Splint-Long | 9002-2 | | |
| Reduction with Local Block | 2009-1 | | | C.P. Resuscitation | 4368001-3 | | | Leg Splint Thomas | 9003-1 | | |
| Chest Tube | 2010-5 | | | IPPB Treatment | 4368002-1 | | | Richard Wrist Splint | 9004-9 | | |
| Shoulder Reduction | 2011-3 | | | Other Specify | 5009-8 | | | **SLINGS** | | | |
| Cut Down | 2012-1 | | | | | | | Zimmer Sling | 9005-7 | | |
| Tracheostomy | 2013-0 | | | | | | | Sling | 9006-5 | | |
| Monitoring | 2014-8 | | | **MEDICAL SUPPLIES** | | | | **CASTS** | | | |
| Minor Surgery | 2015-6 | | | | 3005-4 | | | Arm Cast-Short | 9007-3 | | |
| **DRESSINGS** | | | | **ROOM FEES** | | | | Arm Cast-Long | 9008-1 | | |
| Small | 3000-3 | | | E.R. Observation | 6000-0 | | | Body Cast | 9009-0 | | |
| Medium | 3001-1 | | | | | | | Gelo Cast | 9010-3 | | |
| Large | 3002-0 | | | | | | | Leg Cast-Short | 9011-1 | | |
| Extensive | 3003-8 | | | **SOLUTIONS** | | | | Leg Cast-Long | 9012-0 | | |
| Other Specify | 3004-6 | | | Solution & Supplies | 7000-5 | | | Posterior Mold | 9013-8 | | |
| **EXAMINATIONS** | | | | **DRUGS** | | | | Cylinder Cast | 9014-6 | | |
| Procto | 4000-9 | | | All Types | 4301004-2 | | | Zimmer Knee | 9015-4 | | |
| Gyne | 4002-5 | | | **PROFESSIONAL FEES** | 379 | | | Richard Shoulder Immob. | 9016-2 | | |
| | | | | | | | | Clavical Straps | 9017-1 | | |
| | | | | | | | | Other Specify | 9018-9 | | |

PATIENT NO.

☐ OTHER SERVICES   ☐ X-RAY   ☐ LABORATORY   ☐ PT

DATE _____   RECEIVED FROM _____ $ _____

FOR PAYMENT OF _____

SIGNATURE OF
HOSPITAL REPRESENTATIVE _____

PAYMENT OF THE CHARGES LISTED ABOVE CONSTITUTE ONLY THOSE SERVICES RENDERED BY EMERGENCY ROOM PERSONNEL. ANY CHARGES ACCRUED IN X-RAY, LAB, EKG, OR OTHER ANCILLARY DEPARTMENTS ARE NOT INCLUDED AND YOU WILL BE BILLED LATER FOR THOSE CHARGES UNLESS PAYMENT IS MADE ON DATE OF SERVICE.

**DATA PROCESSING COPY**

Figure 11B. Example of Emergency Department Registration Form

NOTE: This copy of the multiple-copy form goes to the data processing department.

There are two basic scheduling methods: block and individual. With block schedules, all or a large group of patients arrive within a general time frame, such as the morning or afternoon of a certain day. With individual schedules, each patient is assigned an appointment time. Block scheduling may be satisfactory for outpatient services with small patient volumes or short service times per patient. This system also ensures that a sufficient number of patients are available for clinical personnel to attend. But the patient waiting time and inconvenience associated with block scheduling may necessitate the use of individual appointment times. Such a system usually is appropriate for outpatient services with large patient volumes or lengthy service times per patient.

Registration staff must also be prepared to either assist with or completely coordinate the admission of ambulatory patients into the hospital on an inpatient basis. This situation frequently arises in the emergency department and occasionally in outpatient services. Often, such patients must be admitted the same day because of the urgency of their medical needs. Well-organized routines must be developed, and close coordination with the inpatient admitting department must be maintained.

The information required for such admissions is the same as that described in the "Admission" section of chapter 3. However, because the time frame available for gathering this information is significantly shorter, greater demands are placed upon those involved in the process. Frequently, contingency measures must be employed, such as telephoning relatives for information or conducting a bedside admission. However, the medical and psychological well-being of the patient must be given first priority. Likewise, undue stress should not be placed upon the patient's family and friends. The administrative aspects of patient care must not subvert the primary goal of providing necessary medical treatment. A suitable balance must be achieved and maintained.

Contingency plans should be formulated for processing patients during mass casualty or disaster situations. The ambulatory care area is frequently the logical screening, or triage, point for determining patients' conditions and needs and may also serve as the point of entry for emergency admissions. Provisions must be made for communication throughout the hospital as well as with patients' family members and the news media. Basic infor-mation must be gathered and disseminated on all patients treated. Patient identification procedures must be established. Usually, the inpatient admitting department will also be involved in formulating these plans and implementing them as required. Coordination between inpatient admitting and ambulatory care registration staffs is crucial under these circumstances.

A formal on-the-job training program supplemented by a well-formulated policy and procedure manual will help to ensure that all registration staff are properly oriented to their duties. A well-organized, clearly defined procedure manual will support the operating systems needed to fulfill the patient's, department's, and hospital's needs.

## LEGAL CONSIDERATIONS

As with inpatient admission, the legal aspects of ambulatory care registration are manifold. Some of the specific considerations are patient refusals of treatment, hospital restrictions on services rendered, treatment consents, reporting requirements, policies for handling different types of cases, responsibility for patient valuables, and confidentiality of information. Because most of the matters presented in chapter 4 also apply to ambulatory care registration, the reader should refer to that chapter.

## LOCATION AND PHYSICAL FACILITIES

The registration area for ambulatory care services should be located near the entrance to the unit for the convenience of patients and for easy identification and control. It may be desirable to consolidate all outpatient services registration within one area. Centralization of this function facilitates the registration and appointment process, requires fewer personnel, and improves billing and charge accumulation procedures.

If physical and operational constraints permit, emergency department registration may also be accomplished at this location. However, depending on patient volume, it may be preferable to maintain a separate emergency registration staff.

Centralization makes possible a single registration per patient for each ambulatory care visit, rather than multiple registrations and assignments of hospital numbers for each service received. For recurring-visit patients, central registration makes possible a single registration for the entire series of treatments. The unit numbering concept can be utilized; patients can be assigned permanent hospital numbers and issued an identification card to use with each visit. Such a system allows for ready consolidation and retrieval of patient records. The inconvenience of continual reregistration is reduced.

With a centralized registration system, the likelihood of a patient's receiving several different bills for different services rendered on the same day will be reduced. Appointment scheduling can be coordinated for all services required by the patient. Charges incurred can be recorded, totaled, and forwarded to the business office in an organized, consolidated manner. If a cashier is located nearby or included within the registration function, a cash collection effort can be instituted. Cash payment can be tactfully encouraged by clerical staff members, who are aware of the importance of timely payment for services provided.

A waiting area adequate to accommodate the usual volume of patients and their companions should be provided near the registration area. As with other waiting areas in the hospital, it should present a pleasant, comfortable atmosphere and include such essentials as an outside phone and rest rooms. It also should be apart from the general traffic flow of primary hospital corridors.

The size of the registration area will depend on patient volume and the number of staff members and functions they must perform. Generally, sufficient work space should be available for one to six employees. When staff functions include handling large patient volumes, scheduling appointments, collecting cash payments, and accumulating charges, in addition to registering patients, space requirements are, of course, greater.

Sample layouts of outpatient services and emergency departments showing the location of the registration area appear in figures 12 and 13, pages 66 and 67. The examples are intended to depict possibilities, not the ultimate layout.

## EQUIPMENT AND SYSTEMS

As with inpatient admitting, technological advances have provided a variety of equipment and systems that can be used to expedite the ambulatory care registration process. Operational needs and staff capabilities must be considered when evaluating updated systems and equipment. As stressed in chapter 6, the most sophisticated equipment will not correct inadequate operating pro-

cedures or replace poorly trained personnel. Even the most modern equipment will not provide an all-encompassing solution to registration problems. However, when adapted to the proper operating environment, these devices can greatly assist the registration process.

Much of the equipment discussed in chapter 6 also can be utilized for ambulatory care registration. Many of the data collection, duplication, communication, and data transmission methods described in that chapter are applicable to the registration function as well as to the admitting function. Photocopiers can be used to reproduce patient insurance identification and other pertinent documents. Equipment is available that can generate and/or assign registration numbers. Imprinting/embossing systems can provide easy patient identification and information transcription capability. Pneumatic tubes, telephones, and remote printers can all facilitate communication and data transmission between ambulatory care services and other departments.

Ambulatory care registration forms must be developed that allow for the capture of the information presented in the "Functions and Procedures" section of this chapter. Multipart forms are frequently used for this purpose. These forms can also be used to consolidate accomplishment of other tasks, such as securing signatures on treatment consents, assignment of insurance benefits, and payment guarantees. Many hospitals have developed business office and/or data processing copies of these forms, which list all routine supplies and procedures used in ambulatory care services and appropriate charge codes. With this design, the person recording charges need only mark the items used. The prices can be readily recorded from predetermined price lists, and the total amount owed is then calculated. A copy of the form is forwarded to the cashier or business office for collection or billing. An example of an emergency care registration form appears in figure 11, pages 62 and 63.

Systems are available that allow for automated charge input and collection. The operator need only insert a charge document and patient identification in the device. Charges can be automatically priced, assigned to the correct patient account, totaled, and forwarded to data processing, the business office, or the cashier for collection or billing.

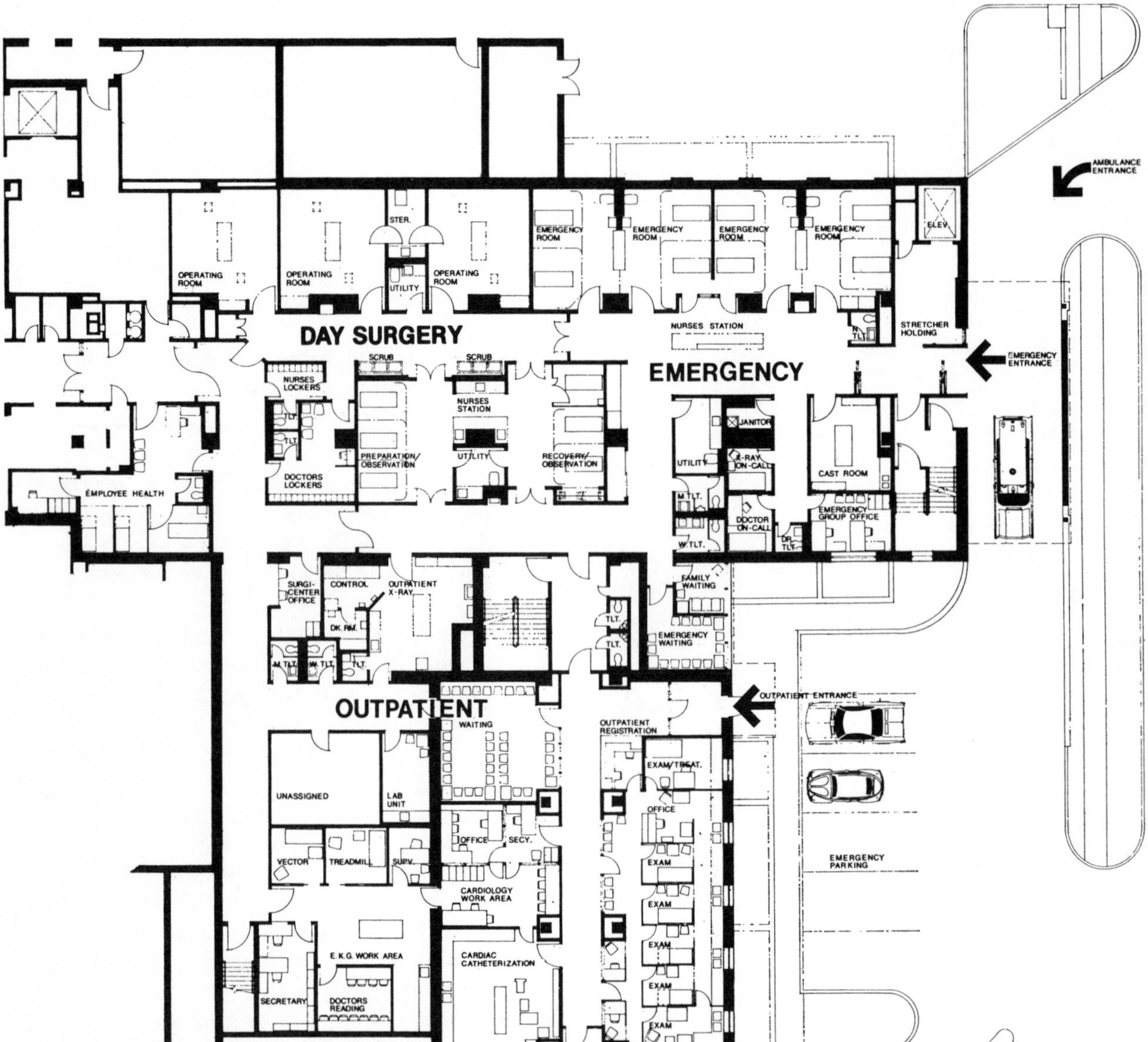

Figure 12. Example of Layout of Ambulatory Care Center

Reprinted with the permission of St. Mary's Health Center, St. Louis, and the Drake Partnership, architects.

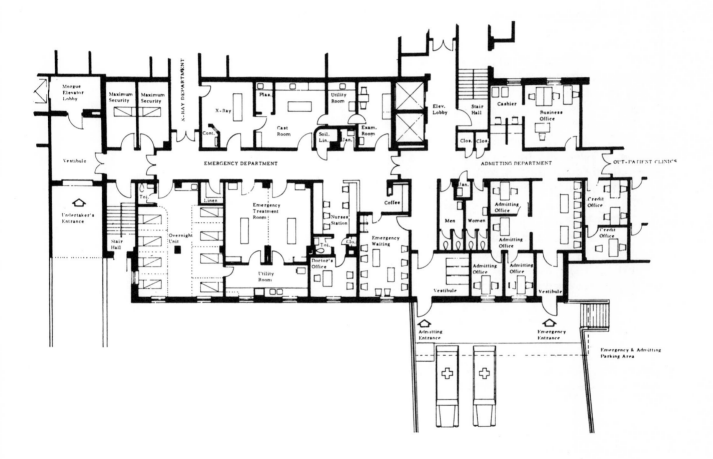

Figure 13. Example of Layout of Emergency Department

Reprinted with the permission of Lynn (MA) Hospital and the Ritchie Organization, architects.

While the patient is being treated in various clinical areas, completed registration documents can be stored temporarily in bins or racks that comprise a location control system. Each individual bin or rack is identified by treatment area. As the patient moves from area to area, his registration documents are transferred to the corresponding bin or rack. Such a system assists with providing information on the whereabouts of patients in large, high-volume facilities. To properly administer such a system, provision must be made for adequate communication between medical personnel and the person maintaining the location control system. An intercom system may be considered for this purpose.

Computerized registration systems have been developed that permit automated data collection and dissemination. The cathode ray tube (CRT), described in chapter 6, is used frequently as the information input/output device. Such systems enable a staff member to register a patient without recording information by hand or using a typewriter. All charge input is introduced via the CRT. The system can be interfaced with the hospital accounting system, so as to automatically produce a bill and record revenue as required. Patient information can be stored for future use. Obsolete information can be purged and updated as necessary for recurring-visit patients. Appointments can be scheduled and revised according to patient load.

# References

American Hospital Association. *Categorization of Hospital Emergency Services: Report of a Conference.* Chicago: AHA, 1973.

_____. *Emergency Services: The Hospital Emergency Department in an Emergency Care System.* Chicago: AHA, 1972, pp. 15-52.

_____. *Management Review Evaluation—Emergency Department.* Chicago: AHA, 1971.

_____. *Medical Record Departments in Hospitals: Guide to Organization.* Chicago: AHA, 1972, pp. 19-25.

_____. *Outpatient Health Care—The Role of Hospitals.* Chicago: AHA, 1969.

_____. *Reshaping Ambulatory Care Programs: Report and Recommendations of a Conference on Ambulatory Care.* Chicago: AHA, 1973, p. 22.

American Medical Record Association. *Glossary of Hospital Terms.* Chicago: AMRA, 1974, pp. 10-11.

Joint Commission on Accreditation of Hospitals. *Accreditation Manual for Hospitals.* 1970 ed., updated 1973. Chicago: JCAH, 1973, pp. 73-80, 119-27.

Public Health Service, U.S. Department of Health, Education, and Welfare. *Ambulatory Medical Care Records: Uniform Minimum Basic Data Set: A Report of the United States National Committee on Vital and Health Statistics.* Rockville, MD: HEW, 1974.

Training, Research, and Special Studies Division, United Hospital Fund of New York. *Systems Analysis and Design of Outpatient Department Appointment and Information Systems.* New York City: UHFNY, 1967.

## appendix A

## AHA Statement on Utilization Review and Medical Audit in the Health Care Institution

This statement affirms AHA support of programs designed to enhance the quality of care and ensure appropriate use of hospital care. The Association, in addition to recognizing that hospitals are required by law to conduct utilization review and medical audit programs with respect to patients whose care is financed by Medicare or Medicaid funds, supports the principle that hospitals should conduct these programs for all patients without regard to the source of payment as part of their corporate responsibility to ensure high-quality health care in their communities.

### PREAMBLE

The American Hospital Association believes that the goals of utilization review and medical audit programs should serve to assure each member of the American public that the care he or she receives in the health care institution is of good quality and is needed. Utilization review is important to all taxpayers and purchasers of insurance or prepayment because it assists in assuring them that their money is being well spent.

### POLICY

1. The goals of utilization review and medical audit programs can best be achieved through a process that places primary responsibility on members of the medical profession who practice in hospitals as members of organized hospital medical staffs.

   The comprehensiveness of utilization review and medical audit programs will be enhanced by conducting audit programs for other patient services such as nursing care.

2. The hospital medical staff should have primary responsibility for developing and using criteria for effectiveness of care and for quality of care.

   In the development of criteria for effectiveness and quality of care, involvement of other allied health professionals can improve the compre-

This statement is American Hospital Association catalog no. S011. Published 1975.

hensiveness of criteria and engender cooperation in the implementation of utilization review and patient care audit programs.

3. Any external program should develop its norms and standards based on empirical data collected from individual institutions as well as from other responsible medical scientific sources.

4. Effective utilization review and medical audit programs can be enhanced when the findings from such programs are used primarily to improve the quality of medical care through medical staff educational programs.

These programs, particularly the medical audit, can be used by the medical staff to review and recommend the practice privileges of its members to the governing authority.

5. Utilization review and medical audit programs in hospitals should review services rendered to all patients (inpatients and outpatients) regardless of source of payment.

6. Summary reports to the governing authority on the utilization review and medical audit programs should be submitted regularly as determined by the governing authority of the hospital.

7. In order that hospitals and their medical staffs can maintain primary responsibility for medical practice in the hospital, in order that the hospital can achieve and maintain due care status and avoid retroactive denial of payment and avoid claim by claim review, all hospitals are urged promptly to establish or strengthen utilization review and medical audit efforts.

## appendix *B*

## AHA Statement on a Patient's Bill of Rights

The American Hospital Association presents a Patient's Bill of Rights with the expectation that observance of these rights will contribute to more effective patient care and greater satisfaction for the patient, his physician, and the hospital organization. Further, the Association presents these rights in the expectation that they will be supported by the hospital on behalf of its patients, as an integral part of the healing process. It is recognized that a personal relationship between the physician and the patient is essential for the provision of proper medical care. The traditional physician-patient relationship takes on a new dimension when care is rendered within an organizational structure. Legal precedent has established that the institution itself also has a responsibility to the patient. It is in recognition of these factors that these rights are affirmed.

1. The patient has the right to considerate and respectful care.

2. The patient has the right to obtain from his physician complete current information concerning his diagnosis, treatment, and prognosis in terms the patient can be reasonably expected to understand. When it is not medically advisable to give such information to the patient, the information should be made available to an appropriate person in his behalf. He has the right to know, by name, the physician responsible for coordinating his care.

3. The patient has the right to receive from his physician information necessary to give informed consent prior to the start of any procedure and/or treatment. Except in emergencies, such information for informed consent should include but not necessarily be limited to the specific procedure and/or treatment, the medically significant risks involved, and the probable duration of incapacitation.

This statement is American Hospital Association catalog no. S009. Published 1975.

Where medically significant alternatives for care or treatment exist, or when the patient requests information concerning medical alternatives, the patient has the right to such information. The patient also has the right to know the name of the person responsible for the procedures and/or treatment.

4. The patient has the right to refuse treatment to the extent permitted by law and to be informed of the medical consequences of his action.

5. The patient has the right to every consideration of his privacy concerning his own medical care program. Case discussion, consultation, examination, and treatment are confidential and should be conducted discreetly. Those not directly involved in his care must have the permission of the patient to be present.

6. The patient has the right to expect that all communications and records pertaining to his care should be treated as confidential.

7. The patient has the right to expect that within its capacity a hospital must make reasonable response to the request of a patient for services. The hospital must provide evaluation, service, and/or referral as indicated by the urgency of the case. When medically permissible, a patient may be transferred to another facility only after he has received complete information and explanation concerning the needs for and alternatives to such a transfer. The institution to which the patient is to be transferred must first have accepted the patient for transfer.

8. The patient has the right to obtain information as to any relationship of his hospital to other health care and educational institutions insofar as his care is concerned. The patient has the right to obtain information as to the existence of any professional relationships among individuals, by name, who are treating him.

9. The patient has the right to be advised if the hospital proposes to engage in or perform human experimentation affecting his care or treatment. The patient has the right to refuse to participate in such research projects.

10. The patient has the right to expect reasonable continuity of care. He has the right to know in advance what appointment times and physicians are available and where. The patient has

the right to expect that the hospital will provide a mechanism whereby he is informed by his physician or a delegate of the physician of the patient's continuing health care requirements following discharge.

11. The patient has the right to examine and receive an explanation of his bill regardless of source of payment.

12. The patient has the right to know what hospital rules and regulations apply to his conduct as a patient.

No catalog of rights can guarantee for the patient the kind of treatment he has a right to expect. A hospital has many functions to perform, including the prevention and treatment of disease, the education of both health professionals and patients, and the conduct of clinical research. All these activities must be conducted with an overriding concern for the patient, and, above all, the recognition of his dignity as a human being. Success in achieving this recognition assures success in the defense of the rights of the patient.

## appendix C

## AHA Statement on the Right of the Patient To Refuse Treatment

It is suggested that the following points receive consideration by hospitals and members of their medical staffs in the case of persons who, for religious or other reasons, refuse to consent to medical or surgical treatment recommended by the attending physician:

1. When the patient is an adult of sound mind, a written refusal is recommended to absolve the hospital, the physician(s), and all other personnel from liability, if any, for failure to furnish the recommended treatment.

2. When the patient is legally too young to make his own decision, the written refusal of the parents or the legal guardian, if available, should be obtained.

3. When an adult patient is legally incapable of making his own decision, written refusal should be obtained from someone authorized under law to act for him, whether the authority rests on relationship or personal or official appointment. (By law, a power of attorney generally expires upon mental disability of the principal.)

4. Before obtaining a written refusal of treatment, the attending physician(s) should explain the medical consequences of such a refusal to the patient or other person refusing consent to the recommended treatment.

5. When consent for the recommended treatment is refused, the attending physician(s) should undertake to obtain a consent for an alternative method of management.

6. The hospital and its medical staff should establish a system whereby the attending physician will report promptly to the hospital any refusal of consent to treatment that might in his opinion have probable medical consequences that would be adverse and substantial.

This statement is American Hospital Association catalog no. S004. Published 1975.

7. The hospital should ascertain that its response to a refusal, whether action or nonaction, is consistent with current state and federal law.

The courts and legislatures of various states have placed restrictions on the right of a patient, or someone on his behalf, to refuse medical or surgical procedures. The legal pronouncements among various states differ in important particulars.

It behooves every hospital to obtain legal advice on an ongoing basis as to the hospital's obligation under state law when such a refusal occurs. Otherwise the hospital will be unable to respect the right of a patient to refuse treatment to the extent permitted by law or to avoid or reduce any legal problems to the hospital itself. Such advice should deal with:

1. Both adult patients and minor patients, including those in either category who may lack mental or legal capacity to consent or refuse consent for themselves.

2. The effect, if any, when the probable medical consequences of the refusal to consent are substantial but not necessarily fatal.

3. The effect, if any, of a refusal based on religious belief or any equivalent personal conviction.

4. The effect of a refusal when another authorized person gives a consent.

5. The types of refusal that may be entitled to unquestioned observance, and whether the hospital or the attending physician has any duty to report any type of refusal to an official agency or court or to take other action.

6. Those persons who have a legal right to consent or refuse to consent for themselves or other persons.

## appendix *D*

## AHA Statement against Use of Social Security Numbers for Hospital Medical Records

The use of the Social Security number as the unit medical record number has become a matter of wide interest in recent years and has been proposed a number of times. Although a better numbering system is needed, and the Social Security Administration (SSA) has indicated no objection to use of its numbers by private organizations if the individuals concerned are willing to furnish them, the American Hospital Association recommends that Social Security numbers not be used as the patient identification or medical record numbering system for the following reasons:

1. The SSA will not edit lists of names and Social Security numbers for validity at the request of other users because the SSA cannot use the income from Social Security contributions for such purposes.

2. The services of the SSA available to Armed Forces hospitals and Veterans Administration hospitals are not generally available to nonfederal agencies or institutions.

3. Under the present system, the time required to obtain a Social Security number from the SSA is approximately three weeks.

4. Tests conducted by hospitals in the use of Social Security numbers have shown that as many as 45 percent of patients admitted either do not have or cannot give Social Security numbers at the time of admission.

Hospitals thus would be faced with the necessity of establishing a temporary or pseudonumber until the correct Social Security number could be obtained—this might be well after discharge or never.

When the pseudonumber is used, procedures must be developed for its conversion to the Social Security number, once that number is available. Every sheet or report carrying the temporary number in the patient's medical

This statement is American Hospital Association catalog no. S005. Published 1975.

record must be corrected to show the Social Security number. Thus a dual numbering system would be required on a permanent basis. This would be particularly objectionable when dealing, for example, with blood banking and x-ray records.

5. It is estimated that at least four million persons have two or more Social Security numbers. Until 1972 there was no law prohibiting an individual from having more than one number.

6. The SSA believes that its records include at least one-half million names of persons who have changed their names and birth dates for various reasons, including many who want to cut their ties with the past or obscure their financial affairs.

7. As a result of multiple numbers and erroneous information, the SSA makes approximately 2.5 million to 3 million corrections yearly.

8. Although the use is not widespread, there is evidence that the same Social Security number is used by more than one person. For example, in the past, persons who purchased wallets with sample identification cards assumed the Social Security number shown as their personal number. It is reported that more than 20 such "pocket-book" numbers now exist.

9. A suffix system is used by the SSA for identifying dependents receiving Social Security benefits, so that several members of the same family can be differentiated only by the suffix letter following the number. The dependent's personal Social Security number, where available, may be used for further identification.

10. The use of a universal number as the hospital account record number jeopardizes the confidentiality of patient information by providing easier access for outside parties, particularly hospitals that are on a broad computer system.

11. Patient identification numbers should be as brief as practical: transposition and reading errors are more likely to occur when a nine-digit numbering system is used.

appendix *E*

## AHA Statement
## on Health Data Systems

A health data system, in concept, provides the methods and mechanisms by which health information can be routinely collected from a variety of sources, centrally processed, and translated into indicators of health delivery.

In recent years, increasing health data needs for purposes of program and policy development, facilities and services planning, provider payments, and institutional management have led to a rapid development of numerous health data systems. Although each of these systems operates under the same general concept, there is a wide variation in sponsorship, participants, service areas, and data bases.

The growth and use of health data systems can serve in the best interests of health care delivery. It is recognized that no one health data system can meet all health data needs throughout the country, because of variations in characteristics of geography, populations, health needs, and related health resources. It is necessary, however, for all health data systems to collect uniform minimum information and be able to use this basic information as a linkage to form a state-national network. Such uniformity and linkage are required to permit comparative evaluations, economies of scale resulting from centralized development, and responsiveness to needs for information at different geographic levels.

Recent national activity has been directed toward the development of a series of minimum uniform basic data sets as an essential component of all health data systems. The series as presently conceived consists of several sets of information, each set focusing on a different area of health services.

It is the intent to develop within each set a list of information items and definitions that at a minimum will meet the requirements of a broad range of users and uses.

This statement is American Hospital Association catalog no. S008. Published 1975.

Potential benefits from minimum uniform basic data sets are many. Of primary importance is their ability to provide users with uniform descriptors, precise tools for communication, and mechanisms through which duplication of effort may be eliminated. The development of health data systems using the minimum uniform basic data set concept would produce these benefits and also allow individual systems and their participants to augment the data sets with additional information to meet their needs and objectives.

## DATA SYSTEMS

1. Hospitals are a necessary information component and beneficiary of a health data system because of:
   a. Their spectrum of health services to the community.
   b. Their education and employment of a large proportion of health manpower.
   c. The proportion of the health care dollar spent in the provision of hospital-based services.
2. Health data systems present the means for orderly and uniform collection of information and its translation into an organized and comparative fact base. Contained within this base is the information that, when properly augmented, abstracted, and used, can contribute to the constructive evaluation and evolution of health services.

   Health data systems are and will become even more essential for at least the following functions:
   a. To provide data for quality assurance programs.
   b. To provide data for efficient and economical health services management.
   c. To provide data for health services planning.
   d. To provide data for policy and program development of governmental agencies and nongovernmental associations.
   e. To provide data for determining health services financial requirements.
3. The growth of individual state health data systems is encouraged and supported because:
   a. The necessary and growing variations in health information needs and uses among the states preclude one national health data system.
   b. The effective development and use of a health data system require close geographic proximity to the suppliers and users of information.
4. Individual state health data systems must be developed in conformity to the following guidelines:
   a. Systems must be developed or sponsored through a cooperative effort, involving at least the following organizations, when feasible: hospital associations, medical associations, comprehensive health planning agencies, regional medical programs, state health departments, Blue Cross/Blue Shield Plans and other third-party payment agencies, and medical care foundations.
   b. All systems must be developed around minimum uniform basic data sets.
   c. The method of data input and output of any health data system must be simple, economic, and, where appropriate, avoid information duplication with other systems. A cooperative effort by technical personnel from sponsoring organizations to plan and program a uniform data base and system can eliminate extensive duplication of data preparation and data processing at the health provider level as well as by the users of such data.
   d. In developing a health data system, adequate measures must be taken to protect the confidentiality of the data while maximizing its use. Of specific concern is the protection of the patient-physician relationship, the right of private communication as provided by statute, and the individual's overall right of privacy. Those institutions and agencies providing and using data must be sensitive to the confidential nature of certain types of information, and they have a responsibility to be judicious in the collection and dissemination of such information.
   e. The system must have the capability to meet the overall objectives of its program and to provide for the various specific data needs of the system's participants.
5. Although the concept of state health data systems is supported, it is realized that because of variation in population density it may be more appropriate within certain states to have

metropolitan health data systems. Further, in certain regions of the country it may be appropriate to develop a multistate system. If such groupings are appropriate and do conform to the stated guidelines, they are supported.

## DATA SETS

6. The American Hospital Association supports the concept of minimum uniform basic data sets, as they will aid significantly in establishing standards of measurement and precise tools for communication between participants in a health data system as well as among systems. They can serve as the foundation of a national network of interchangeable and comparable health information.

7. Individual minimum uniform basic data sets should be developed at the national level through cooperative effort, including coordination and advice from state organizations.

8. The American Hospital Association specifically endorses the Uniform Hospital Discharge Data Set recently developed as the first of the data set series. It encourages hospitals to review and consider implementation of this data set, if they have not already done so.

9. Maximum informational benefits to hospitals from participation in a health data system are best realized only by the participation of all hospitals within the system's service area. The American Hospital Association encourages hospitals toward such participation.

## ASSOCIATION ROLES

10. It is recognized that the problems and issues of health data systems will vary at the national and state levels. The American Hospital Association, with the cooperation of the state hospital associations, will represent hospitals on health data issues that are national in scope, including the development of minimum uniform basic data sets.

With regard to health data system issues at the individual state level, the American Hospital Association recommends at least the following areas of activity for consideration by state hospital associations:

a. Assumption of a major leadership role in the development and maintenance of a state health data system.
b. Assistance, especially to hospitals, to assure maximum effective participation in a health data system.
c. Encouragement of constructive use of health data information by all system participants.
d. Expansion of the minimum uniform basic data sets, as developed nationally, to include items of information relevant to state needs.

# appendix F

## Personnel Qualifications and Characteristics

## JOB DESCRIPTION FOR AN ADMITTING OFFICER*

### Job Duties

Makes future reservations for patients, arranges for admission of patients to hospital, and directs and coordinates activities of hospital admitting office personnel:

Determines hospital privileges of physician who is making reservations by checking against a staff list. Records information that identifies physician and patient, type of accommodation desired, insurance coverage, date of admission, and type and date of operation if case is surgical. Reviews list of unoccupied beds and makes preadmission reservations according to type of case and accommodation desired. Frequently forwards admission form to patients to be filled out in advance of hospitalization.

Interviews patient, his relatives, or other responsible individual to obtain identifying and biographical information. Interprets hospital regulations to patient concerning visitors, visiting hours, and disposition of clothing and valuables. Explains rates, charges, services, discounts, and hospital policy regarding payment of bills. May request partial payment in advance. Notifies particular hospital division to expect patient and arranges for escort of patient to room or ward station. If patient is brought into emergency room, secures necessary information from patient, or from relative or person accompanying patient. Assigns bed or, if patient is to be sent home, explains emergency room charges and arranges for payment. Enters information on record book and forwards cash to business office. Explains differences in rates and charges to patients desiring

*Reprinted from: U.S. Department of Labor, Manpower Administration. *Job Descriptions and Organizational Analysis for Hospitals and Related Health Services.* rev. ed. Washington, DC: Government Printing Office, 1970, pp. 102-04.

change of accommodations, and arranges for change. May obtain signature for surgery from legally responsible patients or relatives. Notifies pertinent departments of patient's admission in accordance with established procedures.

Prepares work schedule for department personnel, based on work load and the number of employees available to perform the tasks. Directs subordinates in such duties as preparing admitting forms, room transfers, admitting reports, and maintaining a current bed index of patients in hospital. Reviews completed work for accuracy and returns improperly prepared admitting records and forms for correction.

Interviews and hires new employees and assigns them to various sections of the department. Arranges for on-the-job training for new employees. Requests wage increases, transfers, and promotions for admitting office personnel. Conducts periodic staff meetings to inform staff of changes in admitting office policies and procedures.

Coordinates admitting procedures with activities of other departments. Places patient's valuables in office safe and issues receipt. May place requests for use of operating room. May answer inquiries concerning condition of patient in accordance with regulations governing such information. May notify family when patient is placed on critical list. May contact police in connection with admission of patients classed within police or medicolegal area. In smaller hospitals the duties usually assigned to the credit department are frequently assigned to this job.

## Machines, Tools, Equipment, and Work Aids

Admitting forms, admitting records, personnel records, room index, time cards, work schedules.

## Education, Training, and Experience

Graduation from a recognized college or university is required. Course work should include psychology, sociology, and personnel and business administration. Some employers prefer a graduate nurse.

Usually requires one to two years' experience in an accredited hospital or social agency.

Usually three months' on-the-job training required to become familiar with admitting office policies and procedures.

## Worker Traits

*Aptitudes:* Verbal ability required to communicate effectively with patients, doctors, and hospital staff members, exercising high degree of tact and poise, and occasionally overcoming language barrier. Also required to understand and apply knowledge of medical terminology.

Numerical ability required to estimate potential patient costs, insurance coverage, and financial arrangements in meeting obligations by patient.

Clerical ability required to recognize pertinent detail in reports and to identify errors [of] omission or [in] calculations when reviewing admittance records.

*Interests:* A preference for business contacts to deal with patients, their families, medical personnel, and hospital employees.

A preference for prestigious activities, to direct the admitting functions of a hospital.

*Temperaments:* Responsibility to direct all activities relating to admitting patients and dealing with them, as well as physicians, hospital staff members, and others involved with admitting section.

Independent thinking, to exercise own judgment in determining actions in emergency situations and in maintaining control of room occupancies.

Analytical, to evaluate other information from established criteria, such as interpreting policies and issuing information on room rates and hospital regulations.

*Physical Demands and Working Conditions:* Work is sedentary. Reaches for and handles admitting records.

Talking and hearing essential in giving and receiving information regarding admitting procedures and room assignments.

Works inside. Usually has own office.

## Job Relationships

*Workers Supervised:* Hospital-admitting clerk and hospital guide.

*Supervised by:* May be supervised by controller, associate administrator, or business office manager.

*Promotion from:* No formal line of promotion. May be promoted from hospital-admitting clerk.

*Promotion to:* No formal line of promotion. May be promoted to business office manager or controller.

**Professional Affiliations***

Hospital Financial Management Association
666 N. Lake Shore Dr.
Chicago, IL 60611

## JOB DESCRIPTION
## FOR AN ADMITTING CLERK†

### Job Duties

Interviews incoming patient or his representative, records information required for admission, and assigns patient to a room:

Interviews patient or his representative to obtain identifying information, such as patient's name, address, age, telephone number, and occupation; persons to notify in case of emergency; attending physician; and individual or insurance company responsible for payment of hospital bill. Types such information on admitting forms and obtains patient's or representative's signature. May prepare identification armband for patient. Explains hospital regulations relative to visiting hours, charges, and payment of bills. May store patient's valuables in hospital safe. Assigns patient to room or ward, based on nature of illness and type of accommodations available or requested. Escorts or arranges to have patient escorted to appropriate room. Routes admitting forms to appropriate department.

Maintains index of assigned and vacant beds. May prepare daily census reports of hospital patients. Receives requests for accommodations and makes necessary preadmission arrangements. May arrange for transfer of patients to other accommodations. May answer inquiries concerning condition of patient in accordance with regulations governing divulgence of such information. May perform routine typing and clerical duties. May compute bills of discharged patients and collect payments. May perform duties of cashier and receptionist.

### Machines, Tools, Equipment, and Work Aids

Admitting forms, typewriter.

---

*Since this job description was published, an organization of admitting managers was formed: the National Association of Hospital Admitting Managers. For information, contact your state hospital association.

†Reprinted from: U.S. Department of Labor, Manpower Administration. *Job Descriptions and Organizational Analysis for Hospitals and Related Health Services.* rev. ed. Washington, DC: Government Printing Office, 1970, pp. 115-16.

### Education, Training, and Experience

High school graduation with courses in English and typing required.

Some experience as a receptionist is preferred; however, most employers will accept an entry level applicant if he can type and shows an aptitude for clerical work.

One to two months' on-the-job training is usually required to attain adequate job proficiency.

### Worker Traits

*Aptitudes:* Verbal ability required to comprehend written instructions regarding admitting procedures and various hospital forms and to interview patients.

Clerical ability required to avoid perceptual errors when completing insurance forms and other documents.

*Interests:* Preference for activities involving business contacts, to elicit and compile personal information for completing hospital forms.

Preference for communication of ideas, to give information to patients, medical personnel, insurance company representatives, and other interested parties.

*Temperaments:* Tact and understanding to deal with patients and medical personnel to admit hospital patients.

Able to evaluate information against judgmental criteria in interviewing hospital patients.

*Physical Demands and Working Conditions:* Work is sedentary. Reaching and handling are required to process various forms.

Fingers keys of typewriter when typing.

Talking and hearing are required to interview patients.

Near visual acuity required to type and read forms.

Works inside.

### Job Relationships

*Workers Supervised:* None.
*Supervised by:* Admitting officer, associate administrator, controller, or business office manager.
*Promotion from:* No formal line of promotion. This may be an entry job.
*Promotion to:* No formal line of promotion. May be promoted to admitting officer.

### Professional Affiliations

None.

## AHA HEALTH CAREERS SERIES: HOSPITAL ADMITTING OFFICER*

The admitting office is frequently referred to as the nerve center of the hospital, because of the increasing scope and complexity of this department. It is charged with governing the flow of patients in and out of the hospital in accordance with hospital policies, serving as a screening point through which all patients must pass.

Vital to the success of the admitting office is the *admitting officer*, who may be male or female. In his key position, he can do a great deal to create and maintain understanding and cooperation between the hospital and the community. Patients, relatives, visitors, physicians, and hospital personnel all have contact with him. The reaction of these persons to the hospital is affected by the manner in which they are treated by the admitting officer.

The admitting officer arranges the admittance of the patient to the hospital; interviews the patient or relative for necessary information; and explains rates, charges, services, discounts, and hospital policy regarding payment of bills. He assigns rooms, notifies the appropriate hospital departments of the patient's admittance, and arranges escort service to the patient's room. He also prepares and maintains records of admittance, transfer, and discharge.

The hospital admitting officer must have supervisory ability, since he is responsible for the efficient functioning of the admitting office and its staff, which may include *an assistant admitting officer* and one or more *admitting clerks*. As supervisor, he interviews and hires new employees and makes work assignments. In addition, he arranges on-the-job training of new personnel and coordinates admitting activities with other departments. The admitting officer reports to the controller, an associate administrator, or the business office manager.

Because the admitting officer is generally the first person a patient sees when he goes to the hospital, the officer must be courteous, understanding, and informed about the hospital. He also should have ability to communicate effectively with patients, physicians, and other staff members. Actuarial ability is necessary for estimating patient costs, determining insurance coverage, and assist-

ing patients in making financial arrangements. Because the hospital admitting officer occasionally must handle distraught relatives or apprehensive patients, he must be emotionally stable, tactful, and poised.

The ability to appraise people accurately and quickly is important for the admitting officer. In many instances he must help the patient or relatives of the patient to plan the financing of the hospital bill. At the same time, he must appreciate the necessity for making the patient comfortable and at ease before discussing financial matters with him.

The educational requirement for the position of admitting officer usually is a college degree, preferably with a major in psychology, sociology, personnel practices, or business administration. Some hospitals use graduate nurses in this position. In addition, most hospitals require one or two years of experience in a health care institution or a social agency plus a two-month or three-month on-the-job training period to familiarize the officer with admitting office policies and procedures.

In 1975 the salary of an admitting officer ranged from $8,500 to $20,000 a year, depending on the size of the institution, its geographical location, and the background and experience of the individual. Work hours are generally the same as those of other offices in the community, although some night work and weekend work are necessary.

For further information about a career as a hospital admitting officer, contact the personnel department of your community hospital or the American Hospital Association, 840 N. Lake Shore Dr., Chicago, IL 60611, for the name and address of the health careers information service in your area.

## JOB DESCRIPTION OF A CLINIC COORDINATOR†

### Job Duties

Acts as liaison between the clinic patient and the medical, nursing, clerical, and social service staffs; coordinates the clerical functions between these staffs:

---

*This careers pamphlet is American Hospital Association catalog no. 3345. Published 1975.

†Reprinted from: U.S. Department of Labor, Manpower Administration. *Job Descriptions and Organizational Analysis for Hospitals and Related Health Services.* rev. ed. Washington, DC: Government Printing Office, 1970, pp. 437-38.

Sets up and opens the clinic by obtaining appointment books and requisitioning patients' records. Greets patients upon arrival, checks appointment sheets against patients' cards, and makes sure that the patients' records are on hand and available to the physician. Assigns patients to doctors in accordance with regulations of specific clinics. Has responsibility for making patients' appointment and reappointments. Reviews medical records, recommendations, and referrals for each patient. Relays a variety of information to the patient regarding preparation for various types of examinations and location of laboratory, pharmacy, and other treatment areas.

Makes minor entries in patients' records and fills out forms for treatments, tests, diets, and various other forms that may be used in specific clinics. Checks accuracy of work of volunteers. Assists and guides volunteers in their duties.

Checks doctors' time sheets, computes and compiles statistics for clinic attendance, and tallies the number of patients seen by each doctor.

Attends meetings of coordinator groups and social service committees to discuss mutual problems, review old procedures, and implement new procedures.

### Machines, Tools, Equipment, and Work Aids

Records, appointment books, and office supplies.

### Education, Training, and Experience

Two years of college, supplemented by courses in psychology, social science, and general science, are desirable.

Some experience in dealing with the general public, in either a hospital or office situation.

On-the-job training in coordination of services rendered by the clinic.

### Worker Traits

*Aptitudes:* Verbal ability is required to communicate clearly and concisely, both orally and in writing, with patients and clinic staff. Must understand clinic procedures and routines and have some understanding of medical terminology.

Clerical ability is required to organize and conduct an efficient clinic and to perceive pertinent details in records and statistical reports.

*Interests:* A preference for working with people in coordinating department services with other departments for the best patient care.

*Temperaments:* Ability to coordinate department's work so that all its responsibilities will be discharged in an orderly and efficient manner.

Able to establish and maintain effective working relationships with patients, doctors, nurses, volunteers, social service workers, and other hospital personnel.

Capable of making work decisions in accordance with rules and regulations of the clinic.

*Physical Demands and Working Conditions:* Work is light. Sitting and walking intermittently throughout the workday.

Talking and hearing for communicating with staff, patients, and others.

Handling of office supplies and reports.

Near visual acuity to read appointment books, schedules, and reports.

Works inside.

### Job Relationships

*Workers Supervised:* Clerical personnel and volunteers assigned to the department.

*Supervised by:* Director, outpatient services.

*Promotion from:* No formal line of promotion.

*Promotion to:* No formal line of promotion.

### Professional Affiliations

None.

# Index